Being Ana

"A fascinating window into the frightening and relentless world of anorexia and, equally, young womanhood."

—Katherine Boyle, Veritas Literary Agency

"Ms. Raviv is a fabulous writer and did an amazing job of simultaneously showing how her eating disorder functioned to keep her from being conscious of the underlying issues while in the depths of it, and showing the reader how all of her behaviors, thoughts and feelings were directly related to those underlying issues."

—Susie Roman, MA, former programs director at the National Eating Disorders Association

"Shani's openness and clarity in sharing her experience with anorexia gave my students a unique opportunity to gain empathy and understanding for the living of an eating disorder. I know it will make them better therapists."

—Dr. John Deninno, eating disorder clinical psychologist and adjunct faculty in counseling and health psychology, Bastyr University

"Shani Raviv is a great inspiration to the many millions out there struggling with eating disorders. *Being Ana* is honest, sensitive, witty, brutal, and so much more."

—Graham Alexander, eating disorder clinical psychologist and director of Crescent Clinic Eating Disorders Unit, South Africa

"*Being Ana* is not only an insightful, raw, and thought-provoking memoir detailing a subject most people know little about, it is also a work by an author who understands how to present a difficult subject with humor and aplomb. Even though the book took her eight years to complete, there is an aching immediacy within these pages."

—Leighanne Law, Elliott Bay Book Co.

Being
Ana

Being
Ana

a memoir of anorexia nervosa

Shani Raviv

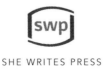

SHE WRITES PRESS

Published 2017
Printed in the United States of America
ISBN: 978-1-63152-139-3 pbk
ISBN: 978-1-63152-140-9 ebk
Library of Congress Control Number: 2017936164

Book design by Stacey Aaronson

For information, address:
She Writes Press
1563 Solano Ave #546
Berkeley, CA 94707

She Writes Press is a division of SparkPoint Studio, LLC.

To my mother, for loving me always.
To my sister, for being a guardian angel.
To my father, for accepting my forgiveness.

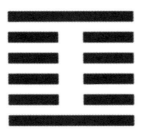

This six-lined hexagram is derived from an ancient Chinese text, *The I Ching*, or *The Classic of Changes*. It is the 27th hexagram, which symbolizes "nourishment"—something that I would eventually desire to guide my life.

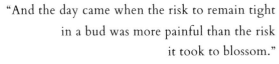

"And the day came when the risk to remain tight in a bud was more painful than the risk it took to blossom."

—Anaïs Nin

Contents

Preface

———

As a little girl, anorexic was not what I hoped to be when I grew up.

And yet, for a decade, anorexia was my path. For a long time thereafter I wished it had been otherwise. I wished I had dedicated those years, and the years that followed in recovery, to feeding the hungry, helping the poor, or teaching the illiterate to read. Something important. When I admitted this to a friend, she said, "Anorexia is about life and death. What could possibly be more important?"

While I was living it, I had no idea what anorexia was about. When I started recovery, I was full of questions: Why did I become anorexic? Where did anorexia come from? Why did I almost sacrifice my life for anorexia? So I set out on a mission to find answers. I needed to make sense of what I had been through. I was desperate to understand why it began. I decided, when I gave up anorexia, that I would work hard to find meaning in it.

Two years into recovery, I was attending a support group for anorexics and bulimics when a woman in the group said, "Please tell us how you healed." I laughed and said, "There is too much to say; I would have to write a book." I was only half serious at the time. I had no idea how to write a book. But I knew I had a lot to say. And I believed in my writing talent. I always knew in the back of my mind that I wanted to write a book, but I never knew it would be a book about my life. In the same way, I never knew that, for a long time, anorexia would be my life. As a teenager, I had dreams. I wanted to become an actress. Make movies. Save the world. Then one day I got lost in a system that backfired on me, and what happened instead was the evil of a starving mind. Although I was never hospitalized, I reached a point where the madness in my head, the malnutrition in my body, and the deprivation of my soul should have killed me. Instead, it took me on a wild ride. I searched for love in promiscuity, happiness in drugs, comfort in cutting, peace in alcoholism, ecstasy in overexercising, and, above all, salvation in starving. I finally surrendered. It took years of therapy to work through the negative emotions that had accumulated in a decade of self-destruction.

During that time I committed myself wholeheartedly to writing and completing this book. A dear friend said to me that some people feel compelled to climb mountains, and that this is my mountain. At the end of this decade-long process, I believe he is right. I worked on the first draft on and off for five years. Then over a period of three years, I wrote, rewrote, and edited many more drafts. Then I rewrote and edited some more, until I finally put my perfectionist tendencies aside and decided to call it complete.

In my third year of recovery, I went to see a homeopath, who asked me a very simple and wise question: "What did anorexia give you?" Without thinking, I said, "An identity, a friend, a purpose, a mother, structure, success, and strength." She answered: "Now you see why it was so hard to let go of it!" It was then that I realized that I had never meant to harm myself. I have since learned that anorexia was, in essence, a desperate attempt to save myself from my overwhelming emotions. Anorexia was never my failed attempt to starve myself to death. That is a common and grave public misconception. Also contrary to the popular belief "once an anorexic, always an anorexic," I believe I am since recovered.

This is a story about my fight to find strength in vulnerability, truth in my identity, and meaning in being me. I have personified anorexia to show that she was much more than a diet gone wrong, a coping mechanism, an addiction, or a girl's vain attempt to perfect her image. I did not just flirt with her as a teenage pastime—she was my life, my vocation, my truth.

I have come through this ordeal with the ability to express my experience of the complexity and nuances of anorexia and to create what is essentially an entertaining narrative about a heavy subject. In it I do not blame society, the media, my dysfunctional family, or my peers for my anorexia. I don't elucidate the role the media plays in perpetuating the cult of thinness because it would contradict what anorexia is really about to me. I was born and raised in South Africa, where I was not saturated with images of "thin." Nor did I grow up in a household of dieters and weight watchers. And before my anorexia started, I was always the thin kid. When it began, no one I knew was anorexic. And I had no idea what it was. So why me? This book answers this question and many more.

Furthermore, I feel that the need to provide an intimate look into an anorexic mind has never been more crucial than it is now. As eating disorders reach epidemic proportions in the United States (and are on the rise in other countries), anorexia nervosa has gained a reputation for being a legitimate psychiatric disorder, not simply (and mistakenly) extreme vanity. According to NEDA (the National Eating Disorders Association), between 0.5 and 1 percent of American females suffer from anorexia nervosa, making it one of the most prevalent psychiatric diagnoses in young women. What many people don't know is that anorexia nervosa has one of the highest mortality rates of any psychiatric illness. Between 5 and 20 percent of sufferers die, especially those whose conditions become chronic. I was very nearly one of them.

A friend said to me once, "If you go through something really painful in your life and survive it, then it's your duty to help others who are going through the same thing." I believe it is not only a duty, but also a privilege. Even though this book started off as a way for me to gain insight into myself and my disorder, it has become much more than that. "This book isn't about you anymore," another friend said to me. For years, however, it was. It was all about me. It was an intense process of developing self-awareness. I healed as I wrote this book.

Now, this project is so much more than just a vehicle for my own recovery. It's a portrait of anorexia, not just as I knew her but as millions know her and identify with her stereotypical, idiosyncratic traits and crazed mindset. I once wrote that if anorexia could be summed up into one line of text on a blank page, the sentence would read: "I don't want to be me." What a sad, hopeless attitude to carry through life. Still, I have yet to meet an anorexic who isn't isolated in her agonizing suffering, who isn't locked in a psychic hell of negative mind talk, who isn't consumed 24/7 with the obsession of thinness and the frightening, insatiable compulsion to starve and overexercise—and the confounding inability to stop.

I wrote this book because I have experienced personally what an emotionally, physically, and psychologically debilitating disorder anorexia is. Anorexics all too often suffer absolute denial in silence, their bodies and minds screaming in pain. This is my attempt to break that silence, to reach out and let people know that there is a way out of the suffering called anorexia.

Whoever you are, whatever you have been through or are going through, I want you to know that you are never, ever alone.

I believe that only by reaching out do we know that others are there. Only by surrendering do we find strength. Only by being vulnerable do we feel human. Only by looking into someone else's eyes do we open our hearts. And, sometimes, only by listening to someone else's pain do we find compassion for ourselves.

This is my story, my offering, my truth.

Chapter One

LITTLE GIRL

Nobody warned me that when I gave up anorexia, I would die.

Nobody told me that the aggressive, confident, wild animal of the night would wake up in the body of a shy little girl who sits indoors and sobs. I didn't know that the person I had been for a decade of my youth would no longer exist. And I was totally unprepared for how lost I would feel after my death. It was the pain of confronting myself as though for the first time, the pain of confronting myself without the identity of anorexia.

I'd be lying if I said I chose anorexia when I was fourteen. I didn't. I just let her in when she had no name, no face, no shape, and she violated me. At fourteen, all I knew when I started cutting out food and skipping meals was that it was a challenge, a test of my willpower. I had absolutely no idea where I was headed —although I knew I was going there alone.

Chapter Two

CLIMBING THE WALLS

I'm not hungry!" I said to my mother as we pushed through the door. The man in the white shirt ushered us in, and I rammed my shoulder into my mother's back as she stepped in front of me. "This way, ladies," said the man. My mother feigned a smile and shot me a look that said, *Don't you dare do this to me now. It is not okay!* and I retaliated with a deadpan face as if to say, *I don't give a shit.* "This is your table, ladies," the man said, pulling the chair back for my mother. "I do hope you enjoy your dinner."

It was going to be a special occasion. It was one of the few times a year that my family came together to celebrate. It was the only time of year that I would agree to go to a restaurant. My grandparents sat next to each other. My mother sat opposite them. I grabbed the seat next to my granny, sat down, and lowered my head to avoid my mother's loaded eyes. My sister sat next to me and placed her hand on mine. My uncle and his wife sat next to my mother. It was going to be a special occasion, and the only reason I was there that night was because it would have broken my grandparents' hearts had I refused to go. It would have hurt them to know that I would rather have been home alone, with my blanket, on the couch, in the company of American sitcom reruns with the sounds of forced laughter and pretend applause.

Instead, I sat with strangers in a strange room and overheard droppings of conversations that didn't belong to me. Knives and forks scraped plates. Forks attacked food. Knives fenced forks. I watched as mounds of food poured out of the kitchen on a conveyer belt of hunger and greed. People chatted and chewed and smiled and threw their heads back in laughter. We sat at a round table laid with its paper napkins folded into little peacock-tail fans and stuffed into glasses. My knife made that serrated sound when I scraped it on my plastic place mat, and my finger stuck to the grease of the embossed lamination bound in a leather folder with the word *Menu* written across in cursive. A dim candlelight was the centerpiece of our small world.

The adults ordered a bottle of red wine. A merlot. For starters, my grandparents would share the soup of the day, my mother would order the mussels in white wine, my sister the grilled calamari, and my uncle and aunt would each have carpaccio. And me, *I'm not hungry.*

"Why don't you sit properly, lovey," my granny said, "and take your fingers out of your mouth. Are you still biting your nails?"

I squirmed around on my seat but didn't change my position. My feet were off the floor, bunched up on my chair. My shoulders were rounded. Both elbows were on the table like I'd claimed my ground and set up my guard. I bit my thumbnail. *I can't stop.* My leg quivered uncontrollably, vibrating the table. My sister put her hand on my knee to stop the shaking. *I can't stop.*

"Good evening, everyone," said a man whose face I didn't care to see. "I'm so-and-so, and I'll be your waiter for this evening." He placed a basketful of thick wedges of warm white bread with crisp crust in front of me and laid a porcelain bowl with scoops of round butter balls beside it. He proceeded to tell us what the specials of the day were, but I didn't hear a word he said because I knew that soon he would be going around the table taking my family's orders. One by one he would write down everyone's appetizers, and once my turn arrived, I would still have no idea what I felt like. *What I feel like.*

I feel like running back to the car and curling up in the backseat and crying myself to sleep. I feel like screaming at the top of my voice that I am here against my will and that I don't belong. I feel like drinking the entire bottle of wine that is set before me. I feel like curling up on my chair and placing my head in my granny's lap while she strokes my hair. I feel like sobbing in my daddy's arms while he holds me tight to stop me from exploding. Shhhhhhhhhhhhhhhhhhhh. Shhhhhhhhhhhh. Shhhhhh.

"Excuse me, miss, what would you like to eat?" said the waiter, turning to taunt me with his gaze that warned me my procrastination would push me over the edge. But he didn't know that I was already falling.

He waited. "Um . . . I'm thinking," I said. He waited. "Um . . . I'll have . . . no . . . I'll have . . . Um . . ." He waited. All eyes were on me, but it was never my intention to steal the moment. My grandfather leaned forward to try to help me decide, but I heard the waiter's clicking pen as he jammed it into his notepad.

He waited. "Why don't I just go ahead and put through the other orders and let you decide," he said. *Decide.*

I have lost the ability to decide. It's a strange thing, that. It's not just that I don't know what I want. It's that I don't know who I am. I don't know what I feel. I don't know why. I don't know anything except that my mind is racing and I don't want to be running this fast. But I can't stop.

"Just make up your mind because everyone is waiting," said

my mother. "It's just one meal in your life. Please stop making such a huge drama out of this!"

She turned to my granny. "This is what I deal with every single day at home! It's exhausting. I can't do it anymore," she said, crossing her arms over her chest and leaning back hard.

"We didn't mind waiting a couple of minutes for you to make up your mind, but I think it's been long enough now," said my granny, who looked as though she was about to cry.

"Just leave her," said my sister. "She doesn't have to eat tonight if she doesn't want to."

"That's a good idea; let's just ignore her," said my mother. "She knows she is ruining it for everybody with that miserable face of hers, and of course I'll be the one she blames for all of this when we get home."

My mother had a way of shutting everybody up while turning the attention on me and away from me at the same time. The wolves backed off, and appetizers arrived. My grandfather opened the bottle of wine and poured an equal amount for every adult as they raised their glasses for a toast. My sister poured her soda into a wine glass. I held up a regular glass with water, my third since we arrived, and chewed on ice.

"*L'chaim!* To life!" said my mother. She clinked her glass hard and had a couple of sips before the toast was over.

"Happy fortieth anniversary, Mom and Dad!" said my uncle. "May you have many more. I wish you long life for the next forty years!"

"Happy anniversary!" my sister said, getting up to hug both of my grandparents. I stood up to do the same.

"You are skin and bone," my granny said, hugging me. "Aren't you eating?"

I saw the confusion in her eyes as she leaned back from the embrace, but I had no answers.

"Leave her, dear, she'll come round," my grandfather said, hugging me.

I pulled away, and he caught my hand gently and said, "We have faith in you."

I sat down again. Everyone ate and talked about South African politics and the near end of apartheid, about my mother's art career, my sister's high school exams, my uncle and aunt's travels and medical careers. But nobody mentioned my sixteenth birthday coming up. I was not a part of the conversation. I tapped my fork on the plastic place mat. I chewed my nails. I chewed ice. I drank my water. I tore my blood-red napkin into tiny pieces and arranged them one by one in a perfect line around the edge of my white plate.

"Don't you want to taste our soup?" my granny said. "Oh, go on. I'm sure you'll like it."

I shook my head no. *I'm not hungry.*

"Don't be like that, it's only good for you!"

"Don't push her, dear," my grandfather said. "She'll come round."

"She just needs to be in her own space," my sister said. "She's fine."

The waiter was back to clear the plates and take orders for the main course. My grandparents debated whether to share the braised oxtail in red wine or the slow-roasted lamb shank. My mother ordered the lamb chops on the grill, as usual, with creamed spinach and pumpkin on the side. My sister ordered the veal in lemon butter. My uncle ordered the venison, which he said was the only real meat because it had been allowed to run wild. But it was his wife who riled me up the most because she had this way of ordering her meals time and again with unequivocal certainty and never, not for a second, wavering. To me this meant that she knew herself. And I envied her for that. She ordered the grilled linefish of the day with new potatoes and oven-roasted zucchini. The chef's special. Then she folded the menu, put it aside, and joined in the conversation, which sounded like white noise. I didn't hear a word anybody said because I had my own staccato monologue going on in my head that was getting louder and louder:

One bite of bread / only allowed salad / just order salad / must drink water / had an orange for lunch / yesterday a spoon of rice / last night three carrots with mayonnaise / no oil / I'm not hungry / fuck this / I want to run away / sit / sit / pretend you're fine / say you ate a late lunch / I hate this restaurant / fuck the waiter / fuck everybody / why can't I be like everyone else? / what's wrong with me? / had half a banana at ten / had two bites of cheese at eleven / had five grapes or was it seven? / fuck I can't remember / I think it was five / shut up / or seven / shut the fuck up / had two sips of juice / had seven cups of coffee / had two carrots with mayonnaise / had three grapes / or was that yesterday?

All the people at the table were drinking, talking, laughing, but there was no sound. No sound except for the monotonous voice in my head slamming into walls like a blind bird, and all I wanted was to block my ears. But how the hell do you block your ears when the noise is inside your own head? And it won't stop. No matter what.

Sometimes they fussed over me: "But why don't you eat something small?" "Go on, you must be hungry." "I bet you haven't eaten all day." "But you're looking too thin." "How about trying this? This looks nice." "Well, what do you feel like eating?" But my answer was always the same: "I'm not hungry." Then my mother started: "I have been trying to tell all of you for months now that this is what I have to deal with every single day. You just can't get through to her. She has made up her mind. She doesn't realize what it's doing to all of us to see her in this state. You would think, from the way she behaves, that eating one meal with her family would kill her!"

I stood up fast and pushed back my chair and threw my fork onto the table hard. It hit a glass, which made that shrill noise glass makes before it shatters.

"I'M NOT HUNGRY!" I said. I turned around, knocking my hipbone on the back of my chair, and stormed off.

Alone in the restroom I paced up and down telling myself to just go out there and order something. Order the smallest, blandest, most un-fattening thing on the menu. I fell against the wall and collapsed onto the ground, hugging my knees to my chest and trying not to cry. Tears stung my eyes, and I moaned aloud to stop them. I stood up slowly and paced the cubicle back and forth, back and forth, hyperventilating. My throat closed. My neck tightened. I couldn't swallow. I couldn't breathe. My breath was right there stuck inside my chest, but it couldn't get out. It couldn't escape.

I slammed my hands against the wall and screamed inside, begging for it to stop. The mirror . . . the mirror . . . I had to see my reflection in the mirror. But it only showed my body from the chest up, and I had to see my stomach. I grabbed the trashcan in the corner to stand on, but it wasn't sturdy enough. I kicked it aside. I pulled my shirt up and jumped up and down so that I could see my stomach in the mirror. I smeared the skin on my belly over and over like I was greasing a baking tray with butter and told myself that my stomach was still flat. *My stomach is still flat.* I sat on the toilet and tried to pee. Tears streamed down my face. My pee was stuck. There was nothing coming out.

I told myself to get back out there before someone came looking for me.

But they never did.

I am so frustrated because I know this is so fucked-up. I know that I am only at a restaurant trying to choose one meal of my life from a stupid menu. But I am stuck inside my head. And I can't get out. I just can't get out.

I glanced at my face in the mirror and dabbed my wet eyes with toilet paper and blew my nose. I saw a girl with pale skin and fear in her eyes. But I couldn't help her. She was already too far away. It was time to go back out there and sit alone with the agony of indecision.

Once everyone else's food arrived, I was still trying to decide what to order. The waiter was back to ask me for the fifth time what I wanted to eat.

"Have you decided yet?" he said, his eyes locking mine. "An Italian salad. No olives! No dressing! And extra lettuce," I snapped.

By then my mother was trying hard not to stab me with her eyes, and my grandmother was telling me to stop acting like a child, and my sister was giving me that "get over yourself" look, and my uncle and aunt were pretending I wasn't even there. By the time everyone had finished eating his or her meal, my desiccated salad arrived. I poked the lettuce with a fork, bit a piece of cheese, spat it into a napkin, and pushed the plate aside. I got up, shoved my chair away, and stormed back to the restroom to climb the walls because the enemy had attacked and there was nowhere else to hide.

Chapter Three

HAPPY FAMILY,
WEEPING WILLOW

I was born with one eye looking to my nose for all the answers. The questions came later. Minutes after I was born, my mother sat up in her hospital bed, propped her elbows on the mattress, and screamed: "Oh my God! I made a baby! A real, live human being!" Salt puddles collected in her eyes, and her blue eye shadow streaked her cheeks like a slither of sky on a cloudy day. My father ran to the hospital pay phone and called every single person he knew to announce the birth of his baby girl.

The doctors assured my parents that a lot of babies are born with a squint and that if my eye didn't straighten out in a few months, they should bring me in for a checkup. At that checkup, my parents were told that my cross-eye was a congenital defect and was there to stay. My mother wept and blamed herself. She tells me now that when she was three months' pregnant with me, after a routine row with my father, she accidentally crashed her Mini straight into a tree, splitting the front of the car in half, both sides wrapping around to clasp the tree trunk like a lobster's pincer. She says the accident caused my squint. My father, on the other hand, tells me that it was raining, that my mother was late, and that she was driving a Peugeot, not a Mini, which skidded into a tree and got no more than a dent. He also denies any argument.

"Maybe your eye was looking at the traffic light while your mother was looking at the speedometer," he says.

My parents should never have married.

My mother was exquisite. She looked like a porcelain doll from the Renaissance era with her perfect tear-shaped face, sweet smile, and eyes that had the innocence of a child. She grew up in the sixties in Johannesburg's middle-class suburbia during apartheid. She was so sheltered from the realities of the world at large that my mother says she didn't even hear about hippies and the flower-power revolution until it stopped blooming. She grew up in a brick house surrounded by a low brick wall, with a garden full of white daisies and a front porch with paint-peeled garden furniture chained to the wall at night to prevent it from being stolen. My mother was a goody-goody, obedient and ever loyal to her parents. She would climb out of bed and creep around on her hands and knees to find her slippers, as she had been ordered not to walk around without them.

At eighteen, one of my mom's girlfriends asked my mom to accompany her on a blind double date. My mom's blind date, Chuck, arrived that day seated in the backseat of a fire-engine red 1965 Dodge Polara that was so long it looked like a ship had docked outside her house. Up front sat her girlfriend, resting her elbow on the rolled-down window. And next to her sat the driver, who had one hand on the steering wheel and the other on his date's mini-skirted thigh. He honked the horn repeatedly for my mother to come out of the house.

The driver had wavy pitch-black shoulder-length hair and wore a wine-red beret. When my mother climbed into the backseat, the driver tilted the rearview mirror and shot her a smile. He had a gap between his front teeth, puppy brown eyes, olive skin, and a manly beard. Although he was the spitting image of Che Guevara's iconic photograph, he was nothing like the revolutionary. Hours later this suave Israeli farm boy, who spoke broken English and cussed like it was the latest fashion, dropped his date at home first and then dropped off Chuck. He told my mother to climb into the passenger seat, drove her home, parked outside, and asked her out on a date.

Nine months later, they married.

My mother says, "The first time I introduced your father to my parents, he kicked his shoes off at the table and wanted to know if the cookies your granny served for tea were dog food." Hearing this story, my father laughs and says, "I never disrespected your grandparents. But why the fuck wasn't I allowed to swear in their house? I kicked off my clogs because I wanted to rest my feet up, but I didn't want to dirty the coffee table with my shoes. And the cookies were a joke. Everyone knew they looked like dog food."

At a subsequent meeting with my grandparents, in an effort to evaluate his suitability as my mother's potential husband, my grandparents asked my father whether he had ever been to a brothel. He said he hadn't but that he had really wanted to go for a long time. He told them a friend had planned to meet him there but then got delayed, and they never made it. My grandparents were speechless. It turns out that my father had thought the question was whether he had ever been to Brussels, in Belgium. Still, despite such misunderstandings, cultural differences, and the language barrier, my grandparents were simply pleased that my mother would be marrying in the faith, a Jew.

Three years and hundreds of brawls later, I was born. Although my father had originally fallen in love with my mother's innocence and she with his wild spirit, her naïveté soon became his source of frustration, and his short temper made her with-draw more and more inward. Although my parents' love for one another was there, it couldn't grow because neither of them knew what to feed it. So my mother and father grew apart from each other, separated by the latent love into which I was born. My mother tells me that my father once said to her, "If you want someone to love, have a baby." He denies her memory. In the story of my life there is always my mother's wild imagination and hyperboles and my father's emotional detachment and rationale. My past is full of contradictory anecdotes, the reality of which I can only guess at.

My mother also says that I was born a few days early. My father says I was born a few days late. My mother tells me that a week before my birth, she was at the gynecologist for a checkup and was told that I was in the breech position, so the doctor reached in to turn me around a full 180 degrees. At the following appointment, he told her the umbilical cord was coiled around my neck. She needed to be admitted immediately for an emergency induction. On the way to the maternity ward she called my dad to tell him to race home to pack her hospital bag because by sunrise they would have a baby.

Whenever I repeat the story of my birth, I mistakenly refer to the umbilical cord as a noose. So as the story goes, I was upside down, manually rotated, strangled by a noose, and forced out unnaturally when I wasn't quite ready to leave. This sounds like me. It wasn't an easy birth, and from the start it hasn't proved to be an easy life.

I was a few weeks old when my mother gave up trying to breastfeed me because she says nothing was coming out and that it was too painful, so she put me on formula. Both my mother and father took turns feeding me a bottle. At a few months old my mother tried to spoon-feed me but says that I often refused to eat.

My mother blames this on my eye. She says she would put me in a high chair and lay down wall-to-wall plastic because as soon as the spoon came toward me, I hit it away. She is convinced that because my squint was making me see double, a spoonful of food coming at me from different directions freaked me out. My father says it had nothing to do with my squint and that I had trouble swallowing and often regurgitated my food. He says there was never wall-to-wall plastic.

Aside from the squint creating a frustrating and confusing world for me from the start, I had various eye problems resulting in poor vision in both eyes but even worse vision in the squint eye. My brain soon enough would choose to ignore the squint eye and compensate for its lack of vision by seeing through my good eye only and so preventing double vision.

I was one and a half years old when I got my first pair of glasses. It was 1977, and the only glasses frames manufactured at the time for children, let alone babies, were hefty, clunky, square plastic frames. Mine were pasty brown and beige with thick, heavy lenses that magnified my eyes. The lenses corrected the squint to a degree, but my eye still needed to gain strength and improved vision if I was ever to use it, which would enhance my peripheral vision. My parents were told that, in order to prevent my squint eye from deteriorating further, they would have to shut down vision in my good eye so as to force me to use my squint eye.

The eye specialists recommended that I wear a patch over my good eye. So I attended preschool with a square-shaped sticky Band-Aid, the size of my fist, over the glasses lens of my good eye. My mother stuck small Band-Aids behind my ears where the arms of my glasses cut into my skin and tiny pads on the nose bridge of my glasses to stop the heavy lenses indenting the skin alongside my nose.

An alternative to the patch was atropine eye drops. Atropine is a highly toxic drug that was used to dilate my good eye's pupil in order to force my squint eye to see. Its side effects can include blurred vision and vertigo; it can also cause difficulty swallowing or breathing as well as delirium or hallucinations. But my parents weren't told any of this. From age two to age nine my mother was told to administer the atropine in my good eye almost every single day.

At the time, my mother, a budding artist, made a living as a children's art teacher, and she tells me that my drawings from early on did not evolve from squiggles to two-dimensional images and later to three-dimensional images as most children's drawings do. Mine did not progress beyond the two-dimensional because of the absence of my peripheral vision, which stunted my ability to make out dimensions and distorted my ability to see perspective.

My mother says I was wild with frustration because I couldn't see properly and that years later, once I learned to write letters and numbers, my handwriting was aggressive and rough. Simple tasks that required writing a number in a block on a page or writing in between two lines were impossible and were a constant source of my frustration and anger. My father says I hated my glasses and that it broke their hearts to see me so uncomfortable and aggravated all the time. But in the same breath he says I quickly adapted to the discomfort, as children do.

I know I felt shame about my eye from an early age. I remember playing leapfrog with my best friend in preschool at age four. I was the crouching frog when my friend leaped over me, accidentally knocking my glasses to the ground. I held my breath in and refused to cry. I was strong. I didn't need help because it would mean that nothing was wrong with me. But still I felt different. I didn't feel pretty because of my ugly eye. I was the only kid with glasses, the only kid whose iris and pupil flew to the side like a circus trapeze act only to hide in the very corner of my eye, and I could do nothing to bring them back to center stage. I picked up my glasses and held the broken frame close to my body. Outdoor playtime ended, and all the children congregated in the classroom. I sat on the carpet away from my friends and held up a gray cylindrical cardboard container over my bad eye as though it were a kaleidoscope. The cylinders were used in those days to package wine bottles. I held it right up against my eye and stared into the dark dead-end void, pretending all the while that I was seeing an explosion of rainbow-colored sequins. I waited that way for what felt like hours until my mother came to get me at pick-up time.

By then my sister had been born. I was just sixteen months old when my mother went into labor on time and my sister slid out like a bar of soap in the palm of a wet hand. The same nurse had cared for my mom when I was born, and as soon as she saw my mother, she said, "Are you back? But you were just here yesterday!" My sister was one week old when my parents were told that she had a hole in her heart. They were soon referred to a cardiologist for a second opinion. There were four complications, all of which were part of a congenital heart defect called Tetralogy of Fallot. She would have to have open-heart surgery or she would not survive.

I know my mother blamed herself for my sister's broken heart. Since her early teens, my mother had suffered from undiagnosed chronic depression, and now her being in a loveless marriage was breaking her heart. By the time my sister was born, my mother's sadness had already swallowed her up, and fear would soon desert her in a place where no one would be able to reach her.

My father knew the facts. They would have to wait until my

sister's body was big enough before the doctors could risk operating. They would have to wait until she turned two. In the meantime, once my sister learned to walk, she squatted every few steps to send her blood flowing to her head so her brain could receive enough oxygen. She wheezed to catch her breath as her lips turned blue and her cheeks flamed red. And during her frequent fainting spells, my father would hoist her up by her feet and flip her upside down to increase the amount of blood that was being pumped from her heart to her brain.

Meanwhile, my mother had chosen the house of her dreams for her family. Before my sister was born, we moved from a tiny apartment in a narrow brick building on a busy main street to a suburban home on a cul-de-sac adjacent to a sprawling park with willow trees and a stream. A big weeping willow sat at the foot of the garden, and my mother dreamed that someday we would play under the shade of the tree and live together in peace and harmony as a happy family. Instead, both my parents worked around the clock to pay for the daily grind, leaving my sister and me at home with a nanny. My parents gradually had less and less faith in their disintegrating partnership.

Even though my sister and I did not share a room—because she had to sleep with a humidifier to moisten the air to help her breathe—we still spent every waking moment together. She was my baby sister, my best friend, my confidante, my other self, and my soul mate. We did everything together, and I nurtured her like a mother.

We sat on the carpet in my room for hours on end drawing and playing make-believe and listening to records. In almost every photo of us at the time, my sister is close to me, by my side, looking at me in awe, touching my arm, hugging me, smiling, and laughing with me. I was the big sister, and when we were together, there was no such thing as loneliness. She was my world.

I remember sitting on my bedroom floor wearing matching nighties and fluffy slippers and watching the record on the record player spin round and round as the needle edged its way slowly toward the hole in the middle. There was one particular record that we listened to that told the story of a toy soldier who only had one leg and was ostracized from the other toy soldiers. Every time we listened to it, I felt a sick creepy feeling inside me. Something scary was happening, and the soldier with one leg was not like the rest.

On my sister's second birthday, she had bright red cheeks and a puffy swollen face, and she was wheezing so much that I had to blow out the two candles on her birthday cake. A week later she was admitted to the hospital to have her chest cut open and her heart stitched up, a procedure she had a fifty-fifty chance of surviving. She stayed in the hospital for ten days and ten nights with my mother by her side at every moment. Each time the doctors told my mother she had to leave, she refused.

She slept next to my sister in her hospital bed every night. Only once did she come home, to wash her hair.

My father remained behind to look after me, although he went every day to visit my sister, leaving me with his mother, who had flown in from Israel and could not speak a word of English. I would only be allowed to visit my sister a few days after the operation because children were not allowed into the ICU. But as soon as the operation was over, my father snuck me into the ICU to see her. He lifted me onto his knee so that I could touch her, and when she saw me, her face lit up.

She lay on her bed wearing a pink-and-white-checked nightie that unbuttoned all the way down, revealing a long scar that ran down the middle of her chest from her collarbones to her belly button. The stitches looked like an elongated caterpillar trudging through sand, its legs bloody and raw. Her wrists were pierced with IV needles, and a bloody bandage covered her belly button. Her jaw clenched as she chewed on her pacifier, sucking in the pain. Her hair was slicked back from sweat. My mother held my sister's hand in hers, pumping her with love while her own spirit was dying. The doctor's words to her were, "If your daughter can walk out of the hospital on her own two feet ten days after the operation, she will make it."

Yet despite the torture of not knowing my sister's fate for those two years, my mom tells me now that the whole ordeal was still not as painful to her as watching me suffer day in and day out, year after year, because of my eye. I find this impossible to believe. I know I suffered. I know that my whole life people have "watched me suffer" to the point of it becoming a family cliché. I know that I focused on my ugly eye until it defined my whole being. I no longer had peach skin, sapphire eyes, silky hair, the sweetest smile, and the most spunk. I had a squint. A deformity. I had something wrong with me, and it was the first thing people noticed.

My sister's scar was hidden beneath her clothes. When we swam or bathed, friends marveled at her scar and wanted to touch it like it was a badge of honor, which it was. She had survived open-heart surgery, a stunning, blossoming, healthy little girl. My "scar," my "mark of shame," was right there in the forefront of everyone's vision, and it was uncomfortable to look at. And my subtle beauty, hidden behind the frames of my glasses, got lost in my sister's pretty shadow.

All the doctors and eye specialists told my parents that I would only be allowed to have corrective cosmetic surgery to straighten my eye once my eyes were fully developed, because otherwise I would run the risk of the operation backfiring and my eye shooting outward in the opposite direction. The operation to correct my squint would have to wait until I was seventeen.

A few months before my sister's operation, my father's brother, who had been working in Rhodesia (now Zimbabwe), was killed in a car accident. My father flew his brother's body back to Israel to be buried. It was then that he decided we would move as a family to Israel in search of a better life for us all and to be closer to his roots. He feared suffering the same fate as his brother, so far away from his birthplace. My mother agreed as long as it would mean a happier life for her children.

My father sold the house with the weeping willow, and we moved to the ground-floor apartment of a small two-story building within walking distance to a main road. We were saving up to begin our lives again. I started first grade at age five and a half. I had many friends and a definite strength of character. Then, shortly after my sixth birthday party, at which I dressed up as an athlete headed for the finishing line, we emigrated. We made aliyah to Israel, in search of a better life for our family, in a place where my parents could be happy and my sister and I could run free.

My mother hoped my father would find work easily and come home for siestas, and my father hoped my mother would settle in easily and find inspiration as an artist to do what she did best—paint. Instead, three months into our new life, my parents' marriage was on the rocks, my father was still unemployed, and my mother was sinking daily, deeper and deeper, into a dark depression. My father took off on his motorcycle every morning in search of work and returned home late in the evenings with no luck. And my mother woke up every morning unable to bathe or feed herself and spent the days staring into space for hours on end, twirling her hair. The medication she was at last prescribed for her chronic depression only made it worse.

For me, however, those were the happiest days of my life. I was in my own world, independent at home and popular at school. I crossed the street to school on my own, arrived home to our apartment on my own, and went downstairs to play with my friends until evening. If there were no photographs of that time as proof that my parents were there with me, I might believe that I was living there entirely on my own, capable and strong, at age six. But there are photographs.

There is one in particular of my sister and me sitting on my mother's lap on a Persian carpet in our apartment. Our ponytails are pulled back, and we both have short shiny bangs. We have happy faces on our T-shirts and are grinning and shrugging our shoulders to our ears and resting our hands on our knees. My mother is slumped like a lump of dough. Her expression is lifeless, like the still lifes she once painted as a teen. Her eyes are vacant, her hair frizzed, and her body fragile, as though she might crumble from our small bodies' weight. Her shoulders are hunched, her chest is caved in, and her arms hang drooping by her sides as though they belong to a puppet with broken strings.

At some point my mother's family stepped in, one after the other, to offer support. My uncle and aunt flew in from travels abroad, and my granny left my grandfather alone in South Africa for the first time in her life. Everyone came to "help out with the kids" while my mother went for checkups at a psychiatric hospital. I remember none of it. The adults decided, eighteen months after our arrival in Israel, without my sister and me knowing, that my mother would travel back to South Africa with us immediately, and my father would stay behind to sell the furniture and the apartment and to wrap things up. Once everything had been settled, he would return to South Africa, and they would make some decisions regarding their failing marriage.

One day, they sat my sister and me down on the rocking chair by the window. My father sat opposite us on a chair, and my mother knelt on the cold marble floor. It was late afternoon, and the air was muggy and hot. My sister and I wore flower skirts, matching T-shirts with rainbows, and buckle-up sandals. Braids hung over our shoulders. Together our parents broke the news to us about our imminent departure. "No, Daddy!" I said. "I'm not leaving."

"But who do you think will take care of you if you stay here all by yourself?" my mother asked.

"I will! I'm even old enough to babysit." I crossed my arms over the rainbow on my T-shirt and turned my head sharply to glare out the open window.

"You're a child," said my father. "You will do what we decide is best for you."

I felt tears collect in my eyes, and I gritted my teeth to hold them back.

"No, I won't. I don't want to go back!"

"You don't have a choice. We are your parents, and only we can decide what is best for you and your sister. It's what is best for your mother. Do you understand that? That's the end of it."

My mother says we left the following day. My father says it was a week later.

On the day of our departure, my mother took us to say goodbye to our friends. Then we packed our personal belongings into our pale blue Volkswagen Beetle, and my father drove us to the airport so we could fly back to our old lives. All I remember is running my fingers along the sleek material and rough stitching of the broken safety belt that hung limp over the car seat like my mother's sad arms. Once at the airport, my mother was so torn between staying and going that she had to be physically forced by authorities on ground control to board the plane. My father knew that she could not stay in Israel a day longer. She needed a bigger support system. He knew she had to return to her parents and her country or she would not make it through.

From the day we fled, when I was seven going on eight, I shut down. I had lost my happiness. And there was no way out. It was the most frightening feeling in the world to be some-where I didn't want to be and have absolutely no power to change it.

Chapter Four

LAWNMOWERS AND
SILENCE ON SUNDAYS

On our return to South Africa, we moved into my grandparents' home in dangerous, depressing Johannesburg suburbia, where I felt locked behind walls and trapped inside fear, confined to the eerie noise of lawnmowers and the dread of silence on Sundays.

For the first few months my sister and I shared my mother's old room, and my mother slept in a single bed in her younger brother's old room. I was placed straight into third grade in my old school, but my best friend from two years before now had a new best friend, and the boys whom I had adored were now older and wilder and stuck to their boy group, of which I was not a part. There was no playtime after school with all the other kids in the neighborhood, as there had been in Israel. There were no kids on our street except for a strange little girl who lived with her geriatric grandparents in a rancid house where they ate cheese fondue. She dared us to stand on the sidewalk and flash our private parts to passing cars. We heard that the neighbor's teenage son had died, and we avoided looking at their house because the curtains were always drawn and it felt creepy.

My mother drove with my granny in her beat-up old car every day to drop us off at and pick us up from school. Every afternoon we drove straight back to my grandparents' house, parked the car, locked the metal gate behind us, and went indoors, where we stayed until school the following day. We spent many an afternoon racing up and down the cement ground in the backyard beneath the washing line, where the drains stank and rotten fruit fell from the peach tree.

My sadness quickly turned to anger that I directed at my mother for ripping me out of the rich Israeli soil and transplanting me to this miserable world coated with an eerie film that left me with a sick sinking feeling in my belly. There was gloom in the air, like the aftermath of an explosion where the blue skies turn gray and the grass gets covered with ash. There was a faint gnawing, grinding feeling that seeped into my pores slowly like water from a leaking faucet. It was the feeling of dread. It was the feeling that my body was being drained. It was a feeling that was beyond my control.

Three months later, my father returned from Israel. We moved to a house up the road from my grandparents' house opposite a public swimming pool with a diving board that was too high to climb. At the house, long shreds of grass crept up the sides of the dirty white stippled walls, and inside the floorboards creaked and the rooms were dark and empty. Our apartment in Israel had been spacious and full of light, and the air had been dense with the scent of eucalyptus trees and fresh cement. Back in South Africa the house smelled of dusty pantry and dank wood, and after school we stayed indoors and watched American TV. When my father was out, my mother put on African music with drumming and gumboot dancing that stomped through the house. It was the one thing that rejuvenated her soul and was one of many things that hammered my heart into my gut.

On my eighth birthday my mother tiptoed into my room carrying a marshmallow chocolate bar with eight candles in it on a tray, singing "Happy Birthday" like it was a birdsong. The winter sun shone into the room, and she knelt down next to my bed and handed me a card she had made me. It was the size of a plate cut in the shape of a heart. The front was covered with a piece of white material speckled with tiny blue flowers. I moved my hand across the card, soft as a baby blanket. It smelled of thick white pasty glue. I turned the card over, and her red writing danced across the page. I felt sick to my stomach. I fell silent. No tears. Just that terrifying feeling. The flowers looked so delicate, like they would wilt from the pungent glue, and the dancing words looked like they would collide. It hurt to receive my mother's love because with it came her pain.

That afternoon my father gave me his card. It was long and narrow and bought at the store. On the front was a cartoon caricature of a fat bald man sitting on the toilet with his pants pulled down to his knees, looking surprised. My dad had written me a note in pen saying he was proud that I was becoming a big girl. My birthday cards symbolized to me, even then, that my world had split in two. I felt it rip. And a year later my parents would sit us down to announce that they were getting a divorce.

Meanwhile, my anger erupted at the most unexpected of times. I remember a day in early fall of that year when my mother was outside standing beneath our huge tree raking the dead leaves while I waited my turn to help. My sister bounded out of the house wanting to rake too. My mother handed her the rake, and I exploded. I kicked my mother's legs and pounded her body. She tried to grab my arms. I lost my balance and fell to the ground. I was on my back in a pile of dead leaves kicking my mother and screaming and crying so much that I started hyper-ventilating and choking. My mother, even with all her might, could not contain me. My father heard us and ran outside. He pulled me up off the ground. Leaves clung to my back, and my shoulders shook each time my chest heaved to catch my breath. I wept so hard that I couldn't breathe. I cried until my eyes burned and my stomach knotted and my throat closed and my body collapsed. He grabbed me by the hand and dragged me to the car. He put me in the front seat choking and struggling to breathe and drove me anywhere he could think of that might distract me from what I was feeling.

Around the time of the divorce, I was finishing up fourth grade, which was in a different building than first, second, and third grade, although it was part of the same school. I was a loner at school in those days and in the years to follow, a pariah of the "popularati." I had no best friend to confide in or group to which I belonged. When the bell rang for break and the other kids raced out of the classroom in pairs, looping their arms, gig-gling and chuckling, I stayed behind at my desk rummaging in my backpack, pretending to be looking for my lunchbox. I stood alone in the doorway of the classroom looking out at the asphalt playground, at the clusters of girl groups sitting in their lunchtime picnic cliques and at the boy groups chasing each other around, shoving one another, and kicking soccer balls against the fence. Nobody wanted to play with the sad girl.

Over the next couple of years puberty hit and my classmates shot up in height; the boys' voices cracked and deepened, and the girls' breasts swelled up and their hips filled out. I developed later than everyone else, and it was obvious, at least to me, that I was going to be the awkward adolescent, the ugly duckling. I grew even more self-conscious about my eye. Even though my glasses had been upgraded to thin-rimmed pink metal frames, they were still large round lenses amplifying my face's gawky features. I hated swimming and gymnastics classes, sleepover parties and school weekends away because I would be forced to take off my glasses and expose my deformity. After school one day a popular girl in my class called me at home to invite me to her birthday party. "Why me?" I said, sure that it was a prank. It wasn't. I think it was pity. I knew I didn't belong in the "popularati," but I absolutely did not want to belong to the "nerd herd" either.

A couple of years later, an incident at school altered the direction of my life forever. That day, all the pupils lined up outside the classroom and, on the teacher's order, marched in to take their seats in desks arranged one behind the other in parallel rows. As usual, the boys scrambled to get the desks against the wall and the girls ran to sit beside the windows. I sat at a free desk where I often sat. It was one of those old-fashioned desks with a wooden slanting tabletop that opened up like a car's trunk so that you could put books inside. The seat was a wooden plank attached to metal that held up the desktop, which was a graffiti mess. Even though graffiti was banned at our school, there were "so-and-so loves so-and-so" in dark red ink, silly jokes in ballpoint pen, and popular adages. I sat down, and the teacher began her lesson. I looked down at the desk and noticed a deep jagged etching in the wood like someone had used a pocketknife. My name was engraved in the desk, and adjacent to it were the words "is a nerd." I felt a lump in my throat. My stomach churned, and my face flushed blood-red. I covered the words with my notebook and fought back the tears. I knew then that I would die if I had to spend one more day in that school being this me that I was perceived to be.

Chapter Five

SCREWED WORLD

Vulnerability was the feeling of being alone and defenseless in my world, but rather than running and hiding from it, first I would fall deeper and deeper into it, and then I would try to fight it.

The feeling started on our return to South Africa and intensified around the time of my parents' divorce. In my parents' twelve years together, each of them had tried to salvage their marriage in their own way. Though my dad still wanted to work it out, my mother said she had had enough. When she told my dad that it was her final say, he disappeared on her, and after a twenty-four-hour search, she found him passed out in our empty bathtub clasping a bottle of cognac. He wasn't even a drinker. They had stayed together a decade too long "for the sake of the children," but the damage had been done to us as a family.

I was ten when the divorce went through. We had moved out of the dark dank house and were living in a generic condo when my parents sat us down to announce it. While my dad sank into bachelorhood and bereavement, moving houses three or four times over the next few years, my mom settled down with my sister and me in a massive, rundown, six-bedroom, two-story house with cheap rent, once again in the same neighborhood as my grandparents. We were no longer mother, father, and two girls; we were now three sisters. My sister and I were prepubescent, and my mother was going through her own kind of post-pubescent transformation from a girly wife to a liberated woman in her midthirties realizing for the first time ever that there was more to life than misery. If my mother had been lost in her marriage, she surely found herself after her divorce.

The house into which we moved was on one half of a double property, the other half of which was a garden so overgrown you would have thought it was a tropical rainforest. It was an anomaly in dry, flat, cemented suburbia, which was why my mother cherished it. It had long itchy grass and droopy trees that cast too many shadows. Spindly branches bent all the way back to the ground to form dark canopies, where my sister and I never dared to venture. In the middle of the garden were stone steps leading down into a sunken hole that used to be a pond and was now dehydrated and home to shrubs, weeds, and a mysterious tortoise that disappeared one day and was replaced by the unexpected arrival of a white rabbit. A long driveway wound its way past two palm trees flanking the facade of the house and ran all the way back to the garage. The back garden had a lemon tree, a plum tree with lilies sprouting at its roots, and a wall coated with scarlet bougainvillea that looked like thousands of entangled paper lanterns. It was my mother's sanctuary. I had yet to find mine.

My mom ripped out the generic kitchen cabinets and replaced them with 1950s wooden units and a round oak wood table from a garage sale. The bathroom, the size of a bedroom, had speckled turquoise tiles that looked like they were coated with a million shards of glass and an old-fashioned dressing table with a defunct built-in beauty-parlor-style hairdryer. The bathroom to me was something out of a horror movie, with the palm tree branches knocking against the windows during storms and the deep bath that you could see if you peeked through the keyhole. Next door was a long narrow room with just a toilet that over the years became our hiding place in the event of a burglary. We figured out a way to climb out the window and down the drainpipes if we needed to escape. But there was nowhere to go; my mother felt like she had finally "come home."

"I just don't know where your mother comes from," my granny often says. My mother was born an artist. She was an outsider in her conventional family and an atypical product of her parochial suburban lifestyle. From the age of five she knew that if she didn't become a tightrope walker, she would become an artist. Paint was her blood. And in time she would defy every art rule imposed on her over the years. She mixed paint with spackle to thicken it. She painted only in oil using warm saturated colors like deep reds, burnt oranges and browns, and black, which was not permitted by her teachers because it wasn't considered a "real" color.

Although her inspiration and inclination to paint fluctuated over the years according to her moods and circumstances, she always painted. Painting kept her alive. Whereas during her marriage she set up her easel in the corner of a room or the garage or attic, she now had the freedom to create the studio of her dreams. So as soon as we moved into our huge old house, she made the whole downstairs space into her art studio. The double doors opened onto the plum tree. Paintings hung on every wall, some her own, some her students', and some of artists whose work she admired. Paint tubes, paint brushes, and bottles of turpentine and linseed oil littered every surface; canvases were stacked against every wall, and her palette was awash with thick colors. Hammers and nails were scattered all over, masking tape hung on door handles, and reams of paper towels were unrolled onto every surface. All her sociopolitical ideas of South African culture, inspirations, and intense creative thoughts were displayed in the magazine images, newspaper cuttings, and photographs taped to the walls. Our home was a living archive of my mother's heart, mind, and soul for everyone to touch and taste.

"You girls have no idea just how fortunate you are to grow up in an artist's studio," she would say. "One day, when you are older, you girls will appreciate it." We would tell her about other kids' families who lived normal lives. "Would you prefer me to be a secretary and go every day to the same office job? And work nine to five every single day? Would you want me to come home and cook the same meals, week after week, and serve tea in the right cups and bake cookies, and make every single day the same old boring routine that drives you to drink?"

In some ways, I would have wanted that. I had attended an elitist Jewish school since pre-school, and I had always felt ashamed to invite other kids into our eccentric, eclectic life because we were so different. The upper-echelon popular kids' family homes were villas behind electronic gates in sprawling lush suburbs. They had landscaped gardens with water features and tennis courts and swimming pools so clear they looked like sparkling mineral water. Their fathers were doctors and lawyers, and their housewife mothers drove Mercedes-Benzes and BMW sports cars. They collected their children from school decked out in the latest fashion, wearing high heels and gold jewelry, their hair highlighted and their nails French manicured. Their homes were painted in pearl tints and had white marble tiled floors. Their lounges had beige leather settees and glass coffee tables with brass legs resting on Chinese carpets. Their kitchens were cut out of homemaking magazines. They had en suite bathrooms, Jacuzzis, and live-in servants. Every room had crystal doorknobs and peach ornaments shaped like Siamese cats. And the parents ruled.

That was not the case in our home. Our neighborhood was ordinary and middle-class, and the wall around our house was unpainted gray cement with a manual gate. My mother drove a second-hand, run-down, smashed-up Golf GTI, which I thought of as a man's car. My mom collected us from school wearing worker's overalls and aprons with paint stains and clogs and striped socks and bangles up to her elbows. She tied cloths around her forehead as headbands and bought flea-market clothing like cargo pants, army boots, purple velvet waistcoats, stockings with frog designs, and red lace-up shoes with green stars. And she only ever wore one earring at a time. She looked young enough to be our older sister and wanted more than anything to be our best friend.

Growing up, my mother's spirit had been stifled by her parents' rigid discipline. My mother's marriage to my father, a charming, hard-hitting hunk of a foreigner, was her first rebellion against her parents' picket-fence mentality, their chaste rules, and Dr. Spock as the family cheerleader. My grandfather was the head of the household, who sat at the head of the table and decided which child would have their turn to speak next. My grandmother was the lady of the household, who served the same dinner on the same night of the week, every week, and told the children to listen to their father and to do as they were told. The family motto of the era was "children should be seen and not heard," and this included not touching or breaking anything, including rules. The furniture and ornaments were to remain in their exact same position and exact same condition at all times.

As an adult in her own right, my mother was determined not to live this way. My mom came alive in chaos and thrived on spontaneity, and she was dedicated to bringing us up in exactly the opposite way to how she was reared. She was never on time, constantly moved the furniture around, and rarely served the same dinners. We had no curfews, no punishments, and we were never reprimanded or scolded. She put no restrictions on anything unless she deemed it dangerous, like touching the electric socket with wet fingers or putting artificial sweetener in our tea or blow-drying our hair because she thought we could get electrocuted. The only things she forbade was our wearing G-strings, because she said it was unhygienic, and filling the bath water up to the max, because the drain would regurgitate rusty dirty drain water. Other than that, there was no structure and there were absolutely no rules.

We were always treated as equals, as friends, as confidantes. We partook in adult conversations and openly expressed our opinions. My mom considered all her friends and colleagues our friends. Not once did she ask for time alone with them or say, "I am having an adult conversation," or, "Go to your room." There was no such thing as, "It's your bedtime," or, "Not on a school night." There were no airs and graces at our house. Our friends never had to ask permission to help themselves to anything to eat or be excused from the table or call my mom "missus." When it was time to leave, they would say, as they had been trained to, "Thank you for having me," and my mother would snap back, "The only person who 'had' you was your own mother!"

Although she taught art at universities and schools and received the occasional child-support money from my dad, she still did not earn enough to survive as a single mom with two adolescent daughters. So she rented out one or two bedrooms to lodgers. There was a bald guy with a moustache who wore running shorts every day and ate only hot tuna from a tin, an Italian woman who let us slip into her long black velvet gloves as she showed us how to hold a cigarette like a lady, and a six-foot-tall British woman who wore a khaki uniform and brought home a black mamba snake that she stuffed into the freezer. There was no privacy; there was always someone around.

For the first few years in that house, my sister and I shared one room upstairs and slept in beds so close together that if we reached out our arms we could hold hands. Once we were tucked in bed, my mom tickled our backs and massaged our feet. "Why don't you take the day off and stay home from school tomorrow?" she often asked. "It's only one day in your life; it won't make any difference." After she kissed us goodnight, she went downstairs to paint until all hours of the morning. We fell asleep to Talking Heads, U2, Van Morrison, and Tom Waits singing us their lullabies.

Our home was a meeting place for young, up-and-coming, politically aware artists. On weekends we woke up to Miriam Makeba's voice singing about human rights and oppression. Her music was banned under the apartheid regime, but my mom's friends listened to it in our home. We lay in the garden, on African sarongs, under the plum tree with the adults, who smoked cigarettes and drank bottled beer and ate avocados and olives. At night they made fires in metal drums and smoked weed and talked politics and art while my mom drank whiskeys straight up and painted. Many of her friends and colleagues were liberals in support of the emancipation of black Africans and were vehemently, if not actively, opposed to the apartheid regime. They were singers, actors, artists, writers, and journalists whose work, like my mother's, was sociopolitical commentary on the state of South Africa in the late eighties, when the government had declared a state of emergency. In those days my mother slept with a silver sheath knife, made by Bedouins, right next to her bed, and once we got a security system installed, she slept with a panic button on the wall above her head.

Still, she wanted us to be exposed to humanity. And we had unlimited freedom, as long as it was within the confines of her world. She took us to gallery openings, fringe theater, and jazz pubs downtown, where we hung out with her alternative subversive contemporaries who drank red wine and played pool. I knew I was privy to a hip scene, an underworld of cool, but I was too young, too self-conscious and naïve to see it as a gateway to a savvy adulthood that would enable me to express who I was. I didn't know who I was. I was just a child with an unformed identity, looking to belong.

My mom had a boyfriend then who was twelve years younger than her. My sister and I came home from school one day to find him splayed out naked on the bed with all his manliness dangling out and his hairy chest exposed. My mom had started a new body of work, and the painting she was working on would eventually, much to my sister's and my shock, be exhibited at one of her shows in a prestigious gallery. My sister gasped and ran out of the room. She didn't speak to my mom for days and refused to talk about it. I had never seen a man's private parts before, let alone so close up, and it wasn't what I had expected to see on my way upstairs to my bedroom. Still, it was nothing out of the ordinary because there was nothing ordinary in our home to begin with.

"It's just a human body," my mom said. "There is nothing wrong with nudity." She practiced what she preached, and I couldn't stand that she often walked naked through the house. For me there was definitely something wrong with nudity, even my own, and my mother's nudity was too intimate for me to accept. I had to walk away. Later on I would tell her, "Close the door when you are taking a bath," and, "I don't want to hug you when you are naked in bed," and, "Knock before entering my room."

She wanted to have open discussions with us about everything. From just about the age we could read, she bought us books with names like *We're Not Pregnant*, complete with explicit illustrations. She wanted us to keep no secrets from her and to always share our feelings. She found it so hard to watch us suffer any kind of pain that she would do everything she could to take it away. But as I grew older, I started to resent that as much as she gave us freedom, she tried at the same time to overprotect us by smothering us with love and sucking away our pain like you would suck poison from a deadly spider bite. She couldn't understand my unspoken yearning to form an identity separate from hers, one that was not based on her needs and desires.

"Why are you so anti-me?" she would ask. I wasn't anti my mother specifically; I was just an adolescent starting to embark on the hunt for my own sense of self. I wanted privacy and normalcy, some regulation, and even some rules. I would come to realize many years later that for me, the type of freedom my mother gave us with open arms was overwhelming and destabilizing rather than empowering and liberating. I didn't want my mom to be so different. *I* didn't want to be so different. Like all teenagers, I wanted to fit in. I didn't want to eat like her, dress like her, listen to her music, or talk about her art. I just needed the space to be me, whoever that was.

Over the years it felt as though there was so much of my mom in that house that I couldn't breathe. Her energy was so big that it filled the whole house and poured outside, sweeping the garden like a tumbleweed in a windstorm. She says she went through major depressions in that house, even one that lasted six months, but I remember none of it. To me, she was always enthusiastic, creative, and energetic. A superwoman. She ran around picking us up and dropping us off, cooking and cleaning, painting and teaching, loving and nurturing. Her energy was larger than life. I could not compete with my mother. And eventually I would make a point not to.

I had just entered my teens when my mom gave me the book *The Road Less Travelled* by M. Scott Peck, and she often reminded me of the opening line: "Life is difficult." She urged me to read J. Krishnamurti's philosophical and spiritual teachings on suffering and Kahlil Gibran's *The Prophet*. She confirmed that life was not supposed to be easy. That it was an uphill battle. But I still wasn't convinced that, at thirteen, it was meant to feel so confusing and intense.

Like many hurt and angry teenagers, I spent hours alone in my room listening to angry or melancholic music, drawing fangs and daggers with blood. A few years before, I had been drawing bubbles and hearts. I discovered the word *existential* and identified myself as an existentialist. To me it meant that I contemplated the meaning of my life and of life itself. I confided my thoughts in journals, hoping to find answers to my troubled existence, and deliberated endlessly on my unknown purpose in this life. But there was an underlying angst that was more than just a teenager dying her hair red and painting her nails black and wearing torn T-shirts that said *SCREWED WORLD* across images of skulls and bones. There was a deep dissatisfaction within. It was an invisible burden. A silent scream. A heaviness. And in time, my dark phase would turn into a black hole that would suck me into it and define my whole world.

At thirteen and fourteen, I remember often struggling with the abstract concept of happiness, of not being able to recognize it as a feeling. I remember making lists of things, small things, to confirm what gave me a sense of satisfaction, but I failed to grasp the actual feeling of it. There was a pervasive malaise, an invasive bleakness that was blocking any connection to that feeling. I understood that supposedly happiness was out there, but I didn't know what it was supposed to feel like because it hadn't belonged to me for a long time. So I proclaimed that there was no such thing as happiness. It was a myth, a lie. I struggled with this a lot. I wondered why the whole world was lying to me about this attainment of happiness. Why was I not able to feel it? Why was I not able to touch it? After a while I stopped wishing and wanting and wondering and just accepted the darkness as my path. It didn't occur to me that there could be a valid reason or even a remedy for this darkness. Life was difficult.

I don't think my mom realized that there was something very wrong with me when at fourteen, I continued to commiserate with her about the pain of life and the fallacy of happiness. She just thought it was normal and part of growing up. Part of it was—the philosophical ponderings and the seeking for truth. But it didn't end there. Something was consuming me. Something was taking me on a journey into darkness, which even I dismissed as the teenager's path to adulthood. I could never relate to the shows I saw on TV where saccharine teenagers floated around their American high schools like bubbles in a fairy tale. My life was not pom-poms and cherry lip gloss and cupid visiting me in my dreams. Throughout high school I was angry and intense, and my life was heavy and confusing, and everything was a huge issue, from the clothes I wore to the music I listened to, all the way to the food I ate. I went through one fad after another in search of an identity. I tried to emulate different people, what they wore, what they ate. I latched onto someone, a friend or a boyfriend, and wanted to be part of their world or their family, to dress like them and eat like them and talk like them. My mother begged me to stop copying everybody and to just be myself. Maybe that was too hard.

At fourteen I asked a friend what it meant to have values. "It's like a list of what you believe, your principles," she said.

"Well, like what?" I asked.

"Like, what's important to you, how you see things, what you value."

I still wasn't sure what she meant. The word *value*, like *happiness*, didn't register for me. The concept was too abstract, and I had no idea where to look inside for the answers, or how deep to drill, because inside I was flooded with some kind of strange pain.

At fourteen my mother took me once to see her psychologist. My mom left the room, and the psychologist asked me why I was there. I sat in her plum leather chair and looked through the drapes at the overcast, still day outside. I felt alone and misplaced, like I was in someone else's story. I told her that I had some kind of problem deciding what I liked and didn't like and that other people didn't have such stupid problems. What I wanted to say was that nothing made sense and that decisions were overwhelming and that everything looked bleak. But I didn't have the words or the understanding to describe that to her. Instead I said that I didn't know certain things, like how many sugars I liked in my tea. It seemed so trivial, even to me. But in retrospect I know that it represented a much larger perplexity, one that was part of a complex and intricate web that had absolutely nothing to do with tea and in essence wasn't superficial or trivial at all.

The session ended, and my mother walked me to the car and tried to put her arm around me, but I brushed it off. "So, how was it?" she asked, "What did she say to you? What did she say was wrong?" I sat in the car next to my mom and crossed my legs in a knot and folded my arms over my chest and looked straight ahead, staring at nothing.

"Nothing," I said in a flat tone.

"What do you mean, 'Nothing'?" my mom asked with panic in her voice.

"Nothing," I said again. I was frustrated with the psychologist because she had no answers and frustrated with myself because I had no reasons. How do you communicate something that you yourself can't even begin to understand?

I wrote down my chaotic thoughts in a black palm-size hardcover book. I didn't call it a journal because my thoughts felt creepy and dark, and a journal was supposed to be something I would want to keep and read again and again. I stashed this little black book in the back of my cupboard beneath piles of papers and books and only took it out whenever I felt the urge to write, hoping nobody would ever find it. A couple of years later, when the little black book was jam-packed with deeply etched black ink and all my terrifying private thoughts, I sat in my room with a friend and told her about it. I told her that it gave me the creeps even just knowing it was there, and that it was full of stuff that I hated and feared. We talked about it for hours, about whether or not I should get rid of it, tear it to pieces and throw it away. I thought that by getting rid of the book, my pain would disappear. But I failed to realize that everything that was inside that little black book was also inside me.

We burned it.

When the darkness came around age eight, over the years I would try to do whatever I could to protect myself from it, and from the overwhelming feeling of insecurity that came with it.

At age fourteen, as a way to save myself from more humiliation, I made the decision on my own to change schools. It was soon after the incident when I saw the writing on the desk. I left the Jewish school to go to a multiracial Catholic coed convent. I had been in the Jewish school for most of my life. It was where Jewish kids went. It provided a good education. My parents never thought to enroll me anywhere else, even though my mom's lifestyle and beliefs were so contradictory to what I had been exposed to there. I chose my new school because it offered speech and drama as a high school major and because it was one of the only multiracial schools in apartheid South Africa at the time. I knew that I wanted to move as far away from rich white spoiled Jewish kids as possible. I hoped that I would finally get a chance to fit in.

I ended up being one of only five Jewish kids in the Catholic convent run by priests and nuns. There were also Muslims, Hindus, Protestants, Catholics, Zulus, and Sothos. It was a multicultural environment where everybody was different. It was somewhere I could reinvent myself and escape the pain of my past. It was maybe even a place where I could finally be popular. I quickly made friends, most of whom came from dysfunctional families and divorced parents like my own. I was finally part of a clique.

Frida was my first and best friend. She was an atheist, and she had been living in exile because her parents were communists. She was born in jail. Her father was killed for political reasons when she was a child. Her brother lived overseas. Another friend, Leah, was born to a Jewish mother who converted to Christianity and became a Jew for Jesus. Leah's father was of mixed race, and her parents divorced when she was a baby. Leah grew up with her mother, stepfather, and adopted younger brother. There was Cindy, whose parents were nondenominational and were going through a divorce. Cindy hid every day in the toilet cubicles to smoke and cry. There was Raheesha, who was Muslim. She grew up with her mother and German stepfather and stepsister and never saw her real father. Another girl, Kim, was from a reputable posh family with a Catholic background, and her father was a lawyer. She acted far older than her years and was highly secretive. There was Benita, who was Jewish, and although her parents were divorced, both of them had remarried, and she seemed the most well-adjusted of us all. And there was Chelsea, whose parents were Catholic Scottish immigrants. Chelsea earned the reputation of being the "go all the way" girl in our clique. She was always smiling. And I was the newcomer to the school. I was the artsy half-Israeli Jewish girl who lived with her wild artist mother in her artist studio house. This was my one shot at a "girl group." And I felt I needed to keep up if I had any hope of belonging.

On weekends we hung out together smoking menthol cigarettes, listening to the song of the moment, and dressing up in one another's clothes. But in less than a year of knowing each other, we quickly evolved from giggly gangly teens lying on the bed with our legs straggled over one another, daring each other to go all the way with some pimple-face in our class, to being sexually active, rebellious, sneaky teenagers who drank heavily and smoked lights. We went from having our parents drop us off at house parties and socials in halls to sneaking out at midnight to catch cabs to the center of Hillbrow, the dingy derelict part of downtown Johannesburg where all the bars, nightclubs, and "adult worlds" were located. It was also at that time that I started stealing, together with Leah. It was small things at first, like silver rings at flea market jewelry stores, but soon enough we were stealing clothes from stores, high on the exhilaration of escape and the relief of not getting caught. The stealing would continue for many years.

Now that I was "cool at school," it could have been the happiest time of my life. But it wasn't. Deep inside I was still the same scared naïve fourteen-year-old with low self-esteem and a major complex about my deformed eye that filled the pit of my shame. My mom had always told me my complexion was like peaches and cream and my hair like golden waves. But I didn't want to be beautiful and sweet; I wanted to be gorgeous and sassy. I didn't want to be blonde and blue-eyed and Jewish; I wanted to be dark skinned and black haired and Indian. I added the letters *Ri* in front of my name to make it sound Hindu.

I tried hard to hide my vulnerability. I dyed my long hair with henna so it turned auburn, and I wore all black to cover my softness—faded Levi jeans, Doc Marten steel-toed lace-up boots, and a leather biker jacket. I sucked on cigarettes that made me choke and drank Sambuca until I passed out, purple-blue and comatose on the bathroom floor. My new friends daubed my innocence with heavy makeup because I wanted to look mature and hardcore. But no matter how much rouge and mascara they packed onto my face, I still looked like a little girl.

Above all, the way we asserted ourselves as young women was through our burgeoning sexuality. At fifteen the girls had all kissed, some a few times and with different guys. Some girls had let guys touch them under their bras, and some even let guys touch them under their panties. I had only had my first kiss the year before, at fourteen, with a sixteen-year-old high school dropout in the body of an overweight man with dirty, spiky blonde hair like a nailbrush. I met him at a teen club. He was a headbanger, which meant he wore angry black clothes with pictures of demons and listened to heavy metal music that sounded like screaming murder. On that night, he said he wanted to show me the view of the city from the roof of his apartment building. When we got there, all I saw were the rooftops of fast-food restaurant chains and an empty parking lot. We stood still, and he held me around the waist. I felt a warm hard throbbing against my groin and a thick slimy thing thrust inside my mouth. It was a moment I had waited for. It made me want to vomit.

In tenth grade there were rumors going around that some girls at school had even lost their virginity. One of the rumors was about Chelsea. The girls were saying that she had gone all the way. Many times. Chelsea was tanned with sleek dark brown hair. She had shapely legs and the figure of a gymnast. Her face was pockmarked under crusty foundation. Her eyebrows were long and dark and curvaceous. Her green eyes were stagnant puddles. And she always had a lifeless expression on her face like her smile was made from a generic mold. But there was something untouchable about her. Even though everyone said she slept around, she didn't care. She wore her attitude like a shield. I used to watch her and think that nothing affected her. It was like her mind was two-dimensional. Like there was no perspective to her thoughts. There was something so simple and uncomplicated about the way she was, and I envied that. I envied that no matter what anybody said about her, she seemed impenetrable. And no matter how many guys fucked her, she seemed impenetrable. I envied her because, in my mind, it meant she could never get hurt.

Chapter Six

DOWN THE
RABBIT HOLE

From as early as I can remember, I had trouble making decisions. It wasn't always that I didn't know what I wanted; it was as though I was looking for guidance from someone who could tell me what to choose.

I remember the day I turned four. It was my big day to be The Birthday Girl at my preschool. I wore a crown and a cutout and colored number four on a piece of string around my neck. I sat at my own table in front of the classroom full of children, who sat before me on the floor in a semicircle. The teacher said to point to the four friends I would most like to sit with me at my table. I knew who my best friends were—we played together every day—yet I could not bring myself to make the choice. So I started from the far right of the semicircle and pointed to the first child in the row, then the second, the third, and the fourth. I look at photographs of that day, and I have no idea who those children are at my table. I don't recall their names.

I also remember that I was petrified of making mistakes. I was six when I lost my first piece of jewelry, a golden abacus on a necklace. It occurred to me then how easy it was to lose something but how hard it was to let that same thing go. I blamed myself. I was seven when my parents bought me my first watch. It was digital with red plastic straps. I bathed with it by mistake, even though I knew not to, and it stopped working. I was angry with myself. I didn't want a new one; I wanted that one. Over the years I became obsessed with never losing anything, never ruining or forgetting anything, and never making mistakes. I was obsessed with getting it right.

With so much self-imposed pressure not to blow it, decision-making was hard. I was five when my first tooth fell out. My mom took me to the toy store to buy me a gift. I was allowed to choose absolutely anything I wanted. Instead, I chose the first toy on the first shelf right near the door. It was wrapped in plastic, and I didn't know what it was. Once I got home and unwrapped it, I found a strangely shaped white plastic thing with a red nose and two rackets that looked like thick heavy bats with holes in them like plastic waffles. It turned out to be a badminton set.

By age six I had formulated a system to alleviate the decision-making stress of getting dressed in the mornings. My plan was to start with the first book on my bookshelf and go through it systematically every day attempting to copy, to the best of my ability, what the characters in the book wore. One day, my whole family was going on a picnic. Everyone was waiting for me to get dressed. We were living in Israel at the time, and it was a hot summer's day, what Israelis call *chamsin*, which is extreme desert heat. My granny had come from the far north to visit for the day, and it was going to be a special family outing, which didn't happen all that often. Everyone was dressed in cotton dresses and sandals, shorts and flip-flops, and they were all waiting for me.

I stood at my closet desperately trying to find something to wear that matched what the little girl was wearing in my Ladybird book. She wasn't even a character. She was the logo; she was on the first page of every Ladybird book. She wore the same outfit in every book: red tights, a navy blue corduroy dress with a long-sleeve turtleneck sweater underneath, and brown shoes with buckles. I had nothing like that. And I hated turtlenecks. Still, that day I was determined to find something as close to what she was wearing as possible. One by one my family stormed into my room.

"Hurry up! Everyone is waiting for you," said my father.

"Why don't you just put on something, anything, something cotton, something light because it's a boiling-hot day and we are all waiting for you!" said my mother.

I was nearly crying from frustration. I just wanted to get it right. I wanted to wear clothes just like that girl. I wanted them to leave me alone with the hard decision that I was facing, standing there in front of my closet. Why was everyone so mad at me for trying to get it right? Eventually, after trying to mix and match T-shirts and sweaters and shoes and dresses, I walked out of my room dressed for the thick of winter, wearing gray corduroy pants and a navy blue woolen sweater that my granny had knitted.

I was embarrassed and ashamed that I had this "thing." I knew my ways were weird. My family knew my ways were weird, but they just brushed it off as another one of my high-maintenance idiosyncrasies. They called me *dafka*, which is Hebrew for *obstinate*. But I wasn't doing it to spite anyone or to prove a point. Every inch of me knew that it was not normal to feel compelled to follow this "system" that I devised in my own head to help me make these simple decisions, but I couldn't stop it. Over the years I confided in friends and boyfriends, and much later I spoke in therapy about the shame I still felt around this, but nobody ever thought to diagnose it as some sort of obsessive-compulsive disorder.

Eight years later I moved from the Jewish school to the Catholic convent, and with the move came the inevitable stress of being a teenager, which called on me to face greater challenges and put me under more pressure to make the right decisions. That was also the year that I first heard about dieting. Nearly every girl in our clique was on some kind of diet, either secretly or overtly. Leah was drop-dead gorgeous with pebble-smooth olive skin, green cat eyes, broad shoulders, and skinny ankles. She dieted. Kim had stick-straight blonde hair and blue eyes, dimpled cheeks, a mature figure, and heavy legs. She dieted. Cindy was curly blonde, blue-eyed, and big-breasted, and she had Barbie-doll legs. If Cindy was on a diet, she was the only one who never made it obvious. Raheesha had dark eyes and black hair and was short and cute. She dieted. Benita, who had introduced me to the school, had big brown eyes, curly brown hair, a huge smile, an athletic body, and strong, heavy legs. She dieted. Chelsea had dark skin, a sexy smile, a curvaceous figure, and shapely legs. She dieted. A couple of years later Chelsea was absent from school for a week. We were told that she was in the hospital having her stomach cut open because she had swallowed her toothbrush. Chelsea was bulimic. Frida, my best friend, was short with a cute round face, a button nose, and shapely legs with robust calves. She was the only girl in our clique who did not buy into the diet hype at all. She loved her body, loved food, and ate whatever she wanted despite the unspoken peer pressure.

I was the new girl with wavy dark blonde hair, tiny half-moon blue eyes and glasses, a narrow waist, a long torso, and long, straight legs. Some guys said I had the best ass, especially for a white girl. Guys were suddenly taking notice of me. I was no longer the lanky teenager I had been the year before. My body had filled out as it suddenly realized I was on my way to becoming a woman: my facial features were proportionate, and my hair was lush. Even my stereotypically beautiful sister with her long blonde hair, olive skin, green eyes, and radiant smile, who was slightly heavier and more curvaceous than me, envied my figure. The girls in my clique told me that everyone said I had The Perfect Body.

I had always been thin. I was eight when two older girls called me "anorexic." I was at a friend's swimming pool wearing a white bikini with yellow string ties and pictures of lucky dice that had faded from the chlorine. I had chosen it although there was an orange one with green frills that I had wanted more. One of the girls whispered something to her twin sister, and they both snickered and pointed at me and said, "You're anorexic, you're anorexic," in singsong voices that sounded like those birthday cards with annoying tunes that turn on and off when you open and close them. I didn't know what *anorexic* meant, but I knew they had said something mean about my body. They ran toward me, one girl grabbed my arms and the other my legs, and they lifted me up like I was a plastic bag with handles and swung me to and fro, dumping me into the water on the count of three. When I popped up again I pretended to laugh so they would think I had enjoyed it. I went home that day and asked my mom what *anorexic* meant, but she didn't know either. That was 1984.

At school, the third graders always peeked into one another's lunchboxes. Most kids had steamrolled sandwiches: two thin slices of pre-cut white bread with a thin smear of lumpy peanut butter or shavings of cheese the color of egg yolk. My lunchbox was packed with four twisted bread rolls like seashells, two with thick wedges of cheese, tomato, and pepper, and two with globs of loganberry jam. Kids teased me about being so skinny and yet eating so much. I ate everything in my lunchbox every day, and by the time I got home, I was hungry for more. I had a fast metabolism and was a growing child.

After my parents divorced, Saturday nights were "going out to the local steakhouse with my dad" nights. Since age nine I ordered the lady's fillet.

"You've got such big eyes," my dad would say. "Have the kiddie's steak, and if you are still hungry we can order more." But I bragged about my ability to eat like a man. "You take after your mother!" he laughed. My mother had a bottomless appetite. She could polish off a one-pound T-bone steak like it was a garnish and still be sucking the fat off the bone.

"I promise you, I could eat another one," she said each time.

And she probably could have. She loved food and stayed naturally slim.

"You are what you eat!" was her motto. My father's attitude, on the other hand, was that food is just fuel. He consumed bags of chips and two-liter sodas in one sitting while watching the game on TV, thinking his body was scoring.

"I don't care what I eat. Food is just there to give you energy one day and then you shit it out the next day," he'd say.

Both my mom and my dad are naturally tall and slender. My mother's weight has remained the same ever since she was a young adult, and my father's weight fluctuated over the years, yet he remained slim. Neither of them ever "watched their weight."

My mom believed in good nutrition. Our refrigerator was packed with assorted vegetables and protein such as grilled chicken, grilled fish, and eggs. We ate butter, full-cream milk, and double-thick yogurt. In the pantry there were anchovies, olives, avocados, whole-wheat bread, carrot cake, and banana bread, as well as chocolate digestive cookies and nut-filled chocolate. Our water bottles were always filled to the brim with ice-cold water. Coffee, sodas, and sugar in our tea were the only things my mother preferred us not to have because we were children and she didn't want us to have caffeine and sugar rushes. My mother never mentioned the word *diet* and had no diet cookbooks, let alone cookbooks of any kind. No diet drinks, no low-fat food, and no lean meat. No matter how she was feeling, no matter how low her depressions or how high her mania, she cooked a wholesome, nutritious meal every night and made our school lunches every morning.

My dad, on the other hand, ate like a typical Israeli. His staple foods were sesame-and-poppy-seed bagels with margarine and cream cheese, cucumber-and-tomato salad with mayonnaise, fried chicken schnitzel, scrambled eggs, and pickled cucumbers. Every few days he bought a cheesecake, cheese blintzes, or an apple pie. And the only meal he ever made in his house was scrambled eggs. When we stayed over at his house on weekends, we ate chips and drank sodas, and if he wasn't taking us out to eat steak at a restaurant, he would order take-out steak hoagies or make us bagels with cream cheese to eat in front of the TV.

Soon after moving to my new school, I hung out with Benita and Kim at Benita's house after school one day, and I was confronted with a crazy concept that up until then had never crossed my mind.

I followed them into the brown tiled kitchen with beige countertops and high stools with plastic seating. Benita took out a baking tray and paper cupcake holders. Kim grabbed a box of cornflakes out of the cupboard. I sat on the counter next to the stove and swung my legs over the side. They bustled around the kitchen and slid around in their long socks, intent on their mission.

"What are you guys making?" I asked.

"Fat-free cornflake cupcakes," they chimed together.

"What do you mean, 'Fat-free'?"

"*Fat-free* means it's got no sugar, silly!" said Kim.

I had never equated sugar with fat or anything other than sweetness, but I also didn't know at the time that this equation was inaccurate.

They mixed the ingredients into a bowl and scooped the mixture into the cupcake holders, using the backs of their hands to brush their hair from their faces. Kim slipped on an oven glove and shoved the tray into the oven. Benita turned on the timer.

"I could never not eat sugar!" I said finally.

"Sure you could," Kim said.

"We wouldn't dare touch the stuff," added Benita.

Then Kim suggested we go to the bathroom to weigh ourselves. The only times I had ever been weighed was at school in fifth grade for a health study and once or twice at the doctor's office. There was no scale in our home and never any talk of "weighing."

Kim, Benita, and I wore our winter uniforms: bleached-white shirts, pleated gray skirts, sheer black stockings, and long gray socks up to our knees. In the bathroom, the scale was set on a fluffy lavender rug the color of an old lady's hair dye.

"You go first," they said. I kicked off my black lace-up shoes and stood on the scale, and the dial flew off to the right, shook for a few seconds, and stopped. It was my first time seeing my weight in numbers. It was no big deal. It meant nothing to me. So I told them my number.

"Okay, now it's my turn," said Benita. Benita told us not to look and blocked our view with her back.

"What do you weigh?" I asked.

"I'm not telling," she said as she stepped off. "It's private."

When it was Kim's turn, she did the same: "I'm not telling either."

"That's not fair," I said, folding my arms over my chest. "I told you guys, and now it's both your turns to tell me."

Kim shoved Benita out the door, giggling. "It's private," they said. They sauntered into the kitchen to check on the fat-free cornflake cupcakes, and I heard Kim whisper to Benita, "Jesus! I weigh way too much, girlfriend."

Benita concurred, "Me too."

What's the big deal? I thought. *It's just a number.* But I wondered what my number meant, where I stood, and how I weighed in according to their criteria. I followed them out thinking about my weight. *Is it good or is it bad?*

At school, the girls talked. And even if you weren't taking part in every conversation, you overheard the gist of the talk, the giggles and the gossip. One girl was on a papaya diet, which meant that was all she ate for a week. Another girl munched apples all day. Another girl ate only low-fat yogurt for lunch every day. The girls huddled together in the classroom, on the playground, in assembly, in church, and there was one word that dominated the girl talk—*fat*. Fat was not just the plump girl in class with chubby cheeks and dimpled knees. Fat was everywhere. It permeated everything from the juice we drank and the sandwiches we ate to our thighs and waists and asses. It lived in food and crawled into our beds at night. Fat was the one thing you did not want in your life. Rather than saying no to drugs and no to sex, girls said no to fat.

My best friend Frida was the only girl who was far removed from the craze. She had grown up in Zambia, where there was no weight-watching competitiveness in her group, and she often traveled to London to visit her older brother, where she was exposed to another world. She moved to South Africa the same year that I joined the convent, and we found common ground in our recent relocation. Frida introduced me to The Rolling Stones and Pink Floyd, Che Guevara and Karl Marx. She had a signed print from Fidel Castro and a bandana with a hammer-and-sickle design.

In the first few months of getting to know each other, like a courting couple, we treated ourselves to falafel dinners on Saturday nights, popcorn at the movies, and lay on her bed eating chocolate bars and listening to The Rolling Stones "I Can't Get No Satisfaction." We had candlelight baths together and discussed what we thought, for hours, about everything from our favorite line in a movie and the different ways in which we each spread jam on our toast, to the effect of capitalism on the proletariat. We watched *Dirty Dancing* over and over again until we had memorized every word and stayed up all night talking about the wrongs of apartheid. We talked about our complexes—my skew eye and her big ears—and styled our hair to cover our "deformities." We filled hours discussing how our asses looked in different jeans and who in our class resembled what part of the human anatomy and whether the school's hot priest was a virgin and the nun a whore. All the while we defined and redefined ourselves according to every little thing that comprised our entire world. And sometime during our marathon discourse, we would pause for teatime. Frida would prepare a pot of Earl Grey, and we would huddle on her bed under a blanket, drinking tea and dunking cookies.

About six months into our friendship, I was at Frida's house one afternoon and it was teatime. "Want one?" she said, tearing a packet of chocolate digestive cookies with her teeth, just like she always did.

"No, thanks," I said, looking down. "I'm not allowed." Frida frowned, cocked her head to one side, and slapped her hand on her hip. She had heard the diet talk at school and knew how invested some of the other girls were in it.

"Not allowed? What are you talking about? Why not?"

"One cookie has half the fat of my daily allowance." I traced the lines on the wood table. I cupped the hot mug with both hands and felt the steam rise to my chin.

"What?" she said, her mouth dropping open and her eyes quizzing me. "What allowance?"

"My daily allowance," I admitted, "of ten grams of fat."

"Oh, right!" she snapped back, staring at me like she had been betrayed. "And who says?"

"I just know."

I have no idea how I "knew" or where I learned any of these dieting "protocols." I must have listened to my friends talk about it. And I know I had started to read food labels religiously. I only remember that these new rules gave me a sense of purpose, focus, and eventually mastery. Down, down, down the rabbit hole I fell clutching my crown—finally I was somebody, I was the dieting queen.

Soon enough, I was as strict with my mother as I was with myself for overstepping the invisible line. I yelled at her if I found her pouring so much as a drop of oil into a frying pan. One night, I heard the sizzle and stormed into the kitchen and grabbed the plastic bottle from her hand and shoved it onto the far corner of the countertop as though it were a loaded weapon.

"What are you doing?" I yelled.

Her bottom lip quivered and she froze, speechless, clasping the pan handle.

"I told you a million times that I don't eat fat!" My jaw clenched like a wrench, and all the muscles in my body tensed up.

"But it was just a small drop," she said, looking like she was about to cry.

"I don't care! I don't eat fat!" After confiscating the bottle of oil, I snatched off the shelf the aerosol bottle of fat-free oil-free cooking spray that I had insisted my mom purchase for me. "You'd better use this; otherwise I am not eating!"

My mother wanted me to eat. She used the spray.

One day, while I was learning to resist the temptation of hunger, I walked into the kitchen when no one was around, took a slice of bread out the package, toasted it, spread butter on it, took a deep breath, and bit. Guilty. I spat it in the trash and tossed the rest of it in and walked away. Seconds later I longed for the toast, walked back to the trash, popped open the lid, and sifted around in the debris. I found it and contemplated, for minutes, whether to eat it. I brought it close to my nose and inhaled the smell of melted butter. Guilty. Guilty for trashing it. Guilty for craving it. Guilty for tasting it. I threw it back in the trash and walked away. *No is no*, I told myself. *No is no*.

If there were a bunch of grapes in the refrigerator and I told myself I could eat three but instead ate four, I felt guilty. Guilty for every bite that was not premeditated. Guilty for every smell that was enticing. Guilty for every envy that was prohibited. The guilt was so powerful that it overrode every other emotion. In time, the guilt would have me throwing my body onto my bed, writhing around, holding my belly as though I had been gutted, and wailing with remorse and regret over giving in to my greed, failing myself. And no matter how hard I would try to always have The Perfect Day in terms of my food, I would feel the guilt every second of every day. It reeked of shame, seeped with disgust, and festered in disgrace.

Ironically, it was my desire to escape the guilt that perpetuated my compulsion to starve.

In time I formulated a more precise list of "can" and "can't" in my head that determined what I was allowed or forbidden to consume. The point is not what was listed but to what extent this list dictated my life. It became my way of life. My manual. My blueprint. But more than that, it gave me false reassurance that my life was under control. I was managing everything because I had this list in front of me telling me what—and what not—to do. The imaginary line in the middle of the two columns was a boundary that I was not allowed to cross. This eliminated the decision-making process because rather than make choices, I knew that whatever did not belong in the "can" column was not allowed. That was final. The list of "can't" continued to get longer and longer and the list of "can" shorter and shorter until the process of elimination was complete. Nobody ever saw my list, even though I would later write it down, but it was always there on the frontline of my thoughts, guarding my insanity.

In the beginning, starving was hard work. It was not innate. Day by day I was slowly lured into another world, a world that was as isolating as it was intriguing, and as rewarding as it was challenging. It was a world that didn't end there. My nature had to change in order to adapt to and survive in this new world.

That summer, despite the fact that I had lost a lot of weight, my mother agreed to let me go to summer camp with my fifteen-year-old peers, after I swore to her that I would eat. I broke that promise as soon as I got there. Mealtime was full of surprises over which I had no control. I faced a predicament where I was forced to make exceptions to my own rules. At breakfast time, when all the teens raced into the dining hall to grab cereal boxes and bread loaves and jelly tins and peanut butter jars, I sat alone, cocooned in my fear. I fingered the plastic package of a loaf of sliced white bread, took out a piece, and tore off a corner, like I was marking a page in a book, onto which I dabbed a blob of peanut butter and jelly the size of the end of a Q-tip. That was my breakfast. Every day. For three weeks.

I tried to get to the showers when everyone else was at the beach so nobody would see me. I heard girls behind me whispering, "That's the girl I told you about that looks so disgusting." Someone invariably walked in on me showering and covered her mouth with her hand like I was a dead body. I wished I could disappear into the drain like my hair that was falling out in chunks. I stopped going to the showers for fear that the girls would spy on me with their friends the next time, that they would peek over the wall to see "that girl."

While everyone else was out there swimming, tanning, making out, playing sports, volunteering, and team-building, I hid in my tent and wrote letters to my mother reassuring her that I was eating. I told her that I ate peanut-butter-and-jelly sandwiches every morning for breakfast. The fact that it was the distorted truth did not mean, to me, that it was a lie. I had convinced myself that this "sandwich" was enough sustenance for the day. And I worked hard to believe it.

Three weeks later, on the train ride home, boys raided the girls' train compartments with shaving cream, and the girls retaliated with their deodorant sprays. Amidst the mayhem there was genuine praise for the sporty guys who had scored the best goals, the caring girls who would later become camp counselors, and the volunteers who helped run the camp. Then there were rumors going around that one boy had the highest score for groping the most girls and one girl had the biggest breasts in the camp and others were the biggest losers and the worst snobs. I was labeled the "concentration-camp victim."

Over the months after my return from camp, everyone

watched my body shrink as though it were being vacuum-packed in slow motion. My school uniform was a yellow dress with a yellow belt, white bobby socks, and black lace-up shoes. The belt was a long piece of thin material with five different holes for the buckle. At my lowest weight my hipbones protruded like knuckle bones under my dress, and I added extra belt holes to the belt but still there was so much extra belt material dangling down that eventually I did away with the belt completely. My shoes were too big for my feet; my ankles were so thin that I wore three pairs of socks at a time and still my shoes would slide off my heels. And my panties were so baggy I secured them with safety pins on the sides so they wouldn't fall down.

But nobody knew that I was always cold no matter how many layers I wore. And that my hair came out in thick wads whenever I wet it or washed it. That I stopped menstruating, but miraculously only for nine months. That at night I lay awake agonizing over thoughts of the day's consumption. That the guilt I carried every day weighed on me like lead. That my hipbones hurt when I lay on my stomach and my coccyx hurt when I sat on the floor. And that the concave feeling in my stomach of dying hunger left in its place an anger that would destroy all feeling.

About six months into my dieting, Frida finally confronted me one day at school. We cut class and headed for the restroom, where we climbed out the window onto the tiled roof, hid behind a wall, and lowered our voices so no one would hear us. We leaned our backs against the hot wall and draped our blazers over our bent knees. The bell rang, and we heard all the other kids racing to their classrooms like wild horses. The heat beat down on us, and we held our hands up to our foreheads like visors to block the sun. We talked about the movie we had seen after school the day before. And then we talked about food.

"I can't believe that Brian stole all my popcorn yesterday!" I said. "Who the hell does he think he is?"

"Come on, it's just popcorn," said Frida. "What's the big deal? Besides, he didn't steal it, he just ate some."

"The big deal is that it was mine! That's the big deal, Frida. You do not just go around stealing other people's popcorn! Who gave him the right to take what was mine?"

"You're only upset about it because it's all you ever eat," said Frida. "The only reason you want to go to the movies in the first place, girlfriend, is so you can eat that damn popcorn."

"That's not true! I eat! I actually would have eaten all my popcorn yesterday . . . "

Frida looked me in the eyes and held her gaze. "You never even bring lunch to school anymore. You used to win the sandwich competitions, but now you don't even make them anymore. What's up with that?"

We heard the toilet flush and someone wash her hands, and we lowered our voices to a whisper. Pigeons pecked around our feet, and the roof slats felt hot and dusty under my hands. I squinted to stop the sun burning, and glittery patterns formed inside my eyes. I felt nauseous.

"Look," Frida said. "If you choose to eat a certain way, then it's a diet. I just think that it is important for you to realize why you are changing the way you eat for some reason or another. I just think it is important for you to know why!"

"I already told you why. I just think that I should be healthy."

"Just admit it! You are on a diet!"

"No, it's not that! I told you, I am just trying to be healthy!"

"There is nothing wrong with admitting you are on a diet —most of our friends are on diets, and they admit it, so why won't you just tell me that you are?"

"It's not a diet!" I shouted. "A diet is to lose weight, and I'm just trying to be healthy!"

"But you know that with all this 'healthy' stuff, you are going to lose weight as well," said Frida, sitting up next to me on her haunches.

"I might, but that's not why I'm doing it."

"Well, I heard that peanut butter is really healthy, so are you going to eat peanut butter?"

I fell silent and played with the sweaty hem on the neck of my blazer. My armpits felt wet and scratchy under my dress, and my bra strap felt too tight across my back.

"Well, maybe it's sort of diet-like because I won't eat peanut butter anymore because it's the most fattening thing in the world. You have to run up and down a flight of stairs six times to work off one peanut."

"Okay," said Frida. "So it is a diet."

"No!" I snapped. I went red in the face and stood up so fast that I felt dizzy. "I already told you that it is not a diet! I just think that I should be healthy, and that is all!"

I turned away and climbed back in the window to the restroom, where I locked myself in a toilet cubicle and tried hard not to cry.

Over the three years that Frida and I were best friends in high school, from age fourteen to seventeen, I got more and more "healthy" until she thought that I was going to die.

On the home front things were worse than ever. I moved to the downstairs room, which had a separate entrance and bathroom, and I locked my door and forbade anyone from entering. Even so, my mother and I had screaming matches every day, with her trying to convince me that "your body needs food as fuel" and me retaliating with "I'm not hungry." But the more she tried to appeal to my rational side, the more stubborn I became in my conviction. My mother made desperate attempts to reach me. Or so she tells me now. I have blocked out most of my memories of her efforts. All I knew at the time was that as long as I was feeling hungry, I wouldn't be feeling anything else.

For nine months my mother stood by, forbidden to interfere, while I starved myself. She had no idea what was going on, nor did I. All she knew was that I had changed. She watched me transform from an innocent, soft, kind, loving girl into a reclusive, vicious, aggressive, defiant teenager. She had lost her little girl. And there was nothing she could say or do to stop me. She knew that if my weight continued to drop radically, she might lose me. But despite all her desperate attempts to reach out to me, despite all the confused letters she wrote to me, the heart-to-heart talks she tried to have with me, the literature on nutrition she had cut out for me to read, she had no way of getting through to me, let alone helping me because, like I did with food, I slowly banned her from my life. My mother was forced to stand by and watch my weight drop and my anger rise. She was witness to my body's physical breakdown, the obvious side that was visible to all, but it was what she could not see or touch that would have revealed the true nature of my disordered behavior.

During this time I should have been hospitalized. Instead, a month before my sixteenth birthday, my father had planned a family vacation to Disney World. He wanted to educate my sister and me by exposing us to another culture—he would take us to New York City, where we'd go to Broadway shows and theaters and restaurants, and then take us south to Florida and treat us to Disney World. Although my parents had been divorced for five years, my mother was going to join us. She tells me that it was supposed to be a special time, with the family together, journeying overseas, and that the thought of me tagging along in the state that I was in was unbearable to her. On the plane ride on the way to the United States of America, I sat in the window seat next to my mother. I wore loose sweatpants and a baggy sweater with sleeves that drooped over my hands and holes at the cuffs where I had pushed my thumbs through. I kicked off my sneakers and lifted my feet onto the seat and hugged my knees to my chest and wrapped my arms around my knees. I was staring out the window when my mom poked my shoulder. The flight attendant asked me if I wanted a breakfast tray. Before I could say no, my mother grabbed the tray. "I'm not hungry," I said. She ignored me. "I don't want breakfast. I said, I'm. Not. Hungry." She ignored me. I put my legs down, and my mother turned the knob on the seat in front of me and my tray table slammed down into place.

Breakfast was raisin muffins with blueberry jam and butter, juice, and coffee or tea. I folded my arms over my chest and bit around my thumbnail till it bled. This would usually be the moment that she would say something. She would remind me that what I was doing was not right, not healthy, and not fair. And then it would be my turn to retaliate with something to remind her that it was none of her business, not her body, and out of her hands. But this time was different. She didn't look at me. She didn't flinch. Instead, she sat dead still and looked straight ahead. Then she spoke in the most deadpan matter-of-fact voice I'd ever heard her use. She said, "My child, if you carry on this way, it would be better for you to die."

The plane landed, and I lugged those words with me every day of my life from that point on.

In America, I started eating. But I didn't just eat. I piled the food on at buffets; I ate tubs upon tubs of ice cream, pizzas, hamburgers, cheesecakes, milkshakes, and sodas. I made up for every starving moment. My parents were ecstatic that I was eating throughout the day. And even late at night, when everybody was getting ready for bed, I was courting the refrigerator, still loading my bowl with more scoops of ice cream, satisfying myself with my parents' approval. But none of us realized what was really happening. It was the opposite side of the same dirty coin. I was still in the grip of the disorder. I was bingeing. None of us realized that overeating was as unhealthy for my body and as damaging to my psyche as starving. I remember feeling like the special child. I had earned my right to indulge.

Three weeks later we arrived back at the Johannesburg airport, and I weighed myself on the luggage scale. In three weeks I had put back on all the weight it had taken me nine months to lose. My father took a cab home, and my grandparents collected us girls from the airport. My grandfather drove with my mother in front and my sister, me, and my granny in the back. I leaned against the door, and my granny told me to sit properly and move away from the door in a voice that was more panicked than her usual panicked voice. She told me not to lean against the car door and not to touch the car door handle and to sit tight. I remember thinking that she was so paranoid.

When we arrived home, she set the kitchen table with teacups and saucers and placed her famous chocolate cake in the middle. I had just sat down when my granny, who stood next to me to cut the cake, put her soft hand under my chin.

"We have something to tell you, my sweetheart," she said. She had a deep frown, and I could see by the lines on her neck that she was straining to speak. Her eyes were hard as glass.

"What?" I snapped in reaction to the sudden silence. She stroked my cheek with the back of her hand, and I felt the smooth cold band of her wedding ring against my skin.

"I am so sorry to have to tell you this, my love, but your friend Kim was in a terrible, terrible car accident . . . and she was killed."

Tears streamed down my granny's face. My mother dropped her teacup, and my sister's face went pale.

"What?" I shook my head to clear the air and clutched my arms over my exploding belly and glanced at everyone's faces to see if it was real.

"We wanted to wait for you to arrive home first before we told you because we didn't want to ruin your vacation," my granny said.

Her voice cracked into hundreds of pieces. I looked up at her and burst into tears. My head fell against her body, my arms wrapped around her waist, and I wept. She held my head in her arms and stroked my hair and whispered, "I know, I know . . ."

My mother came over to me and scooped me up and hugged me and held me. I let her. She sat down and embraced me on her lap like a child, and my tears soaked her shoulder wet.

What I heard was beyond my understanding, and what I felt was beyond anything I had ever felt before. Kim was gone. I had missed the funeral. And when I started school again, she would not be there. Back at school, we, her friends, walked up to one another like zombies and collapsed into each other's arms and sobbed. Our eyes were lost, and our voices were broken. At assembly on the first day back when the principal announced Kim's death, the entire school froze, and that terrifying eerie feeling that I felt over the years was no longer just inside me but everywhere I looked—in my friends' faces, on the playground, in the trees, and in the sky.

And after a few weeks, when the school regained its uniform rhythm, the teachers urged us to do the same and "get on with it." None of them spoke to us about Kim's life or her death.

It was as though she had never existed, while all I could think of was the hopelessness of life, the fragility and pointlessness and unfairness of it all. The teachers returned to their dull lessons; our whole world had changed. Our math teacher taught us algebra—said to be the science of restoring what is missing or the reunion of broken parts—but to me it was just senseless numbers. Our Afrikaans teacher read a poem about a half-man-half-monster that emerges from a dark pond. Our history teacher taught us about the Cold War, and our English teacher taught about a pompous author who died a hundred years before.

I hated them for disrespecting Kim by pretending she never existed and expecting us to be interested in their lessons, which meant nothing to me. I was engrossed by thoughts of death and perturbed by the meaning of life, and I sat in their classrooms fighting back tears and wanting to spit fury. I had far bigger things on my mind than petty grades, irrelevant facts, and meaningless figures. I had loss, grief, despair, and hopelessness.

The person who struggled the most with Kim's death was her boyfriend Tyrone. They had been going out for a year before she died. He was heartbroken and alone in his pain, and he looked to her friends for comfort. We became close and started hanging out together, and we'd spend a lot of time talking about our memories of Kim and what we loved and missed about her. My mother took pity on me and gave me the freedom to grieve and allowed me the comfort she thought that I needed. I was sixteen when my mother allowed Tyrone, a horny, testosterone-driven seventeen-year-old man with stubble on his face and muscles on his body and a deep man's voice, to sleep with me in my single bed. My mom hoped it would offer us comfort in our time of mourning. Tyrone stayed over many nights because his mother knew he would do whatever he wanted anyway. He slept with me in my bed, and we cuddled and cried, and our bodies got hot under the blanket and his thing got hard. I was intrigued and at the same time scared of this bond that was forming between us. I thought it was wrong to be close in this way with my dead friend's boyfriend, even if she was not around to witness it. We talked about it a lot. And we convinced each other that she would be okay with it, that she would even condone it. But I hated that he compared me to Kim in bed. He stroked my face and told me how much he missed her and how beautiful she was and that being with me was bringing him closer to her. He was gentle, but his charm shone like fake gold. He told me he loved me. He wanted me. He held me tight in his big strong arms, and I put my head against his soft T-shirt. It was comforting, and for as long as it lasted, it lulled my pain.

In the first few weeks, he didn't even mention sex, but then he started suggesting that it was the right thing for us to do. He'd put his hand on my neck and say softly that he felt we were ready. "Think about it," he'd say before leaving. I cried every time he left. I cried for Kim. I cried for the pain to stop. I curled up on my bed listening to raw lyrics, my stomach full of hollowness.

I knew that sex was a big deal even if I didn't want it to be and that I was supposed to feel "ready" when it happened, but here he was, offering himself to me. Everyone at school thought he was hot. He wanted me, which meant I was sexy. He liked me and even said he loved me. He had slept with girls before, which meant he was experienced. And if I said yes to him, then I would not have to be the last one in our group to go all the way. I would not be the odd one out.

He came over to my house after school one day. My mom dropped us off and said she was going to the store and would be back soon. I wore my winter school uniform—a navy blue blazer, a white button-up collared shirt, a gray pleated skirt, long socks up to my knees, and black lace-up shoes. We went to my room. We took our blazers off, and without any kissing, holding, or touching, he suggested that we "do it now" before my mom got home. He motioned me onto my single bed, hitched up my skirt, and slid my panties off, and I pulled my knees together. He unzipped his pants and parted my legs, and the next minute this thing was inside me and I felt nothing. I felt no pleasure or pain. It didn't last long, maybe a minute. I was surprised that I felt nothing and that there was no blood. There. I did it. It was over. I would not be the last one. He grabbed an empty tea mug from next to my bed and shot his load into it. As I pulled up my panties and he zipped up his pants, I heard my mother walk through the front door. A few minutes later we strolled into the kitchen to greet her and pretended that nothing had happened.

I had performed the most intimate of acts with no more than silence as my consent. The lack of desire or emotion or pleasure would bury a feeling of violation inside me, which I would not confront until eight years later. I remember a scene I saw in a movie that I watched when I was too young. In the scene, a woman was dancing seductively, and a man pinned her down onto a pinball machine and had his way with her. I remember bragging to my mom's male friend that I had seen this film; he was appalled that I had watched it. I don't know that I fully identified that scene in the movie as rape. But I do know that the day I lost my virginity, I mistook it for sex.

My botched memories of being sixteen and seventeen are filled with reckless abandon. I was an adolescent in high school trying to play the role of an adult in the real world. I had to decide what to do with my life and my future while living only in the moment. I fought hard to claim my independence in the world and to separate myself from my mother, who, at the same time, was desperate to get me to see the perils of my ways. And I tried to stake out some privacy in a household saturated with femininity.

My mother's home had been converted into an estrogen party, a sisterhood of five over-emotional menstruating females and me. My mom's best friend and her two daughters had emigrated from Australia and moved in with us for their transition year. Everywhere I looked I saw panties hanging out to dry over the stairwell, tampons lying in the fruit bowl, and Kleenex soaked with our erratic moods from each of our emotional upheavals. We were six females, each going through her own personal crisis. My mom gunned ahead in her overachieving mania; her friend was a stay-at-home depressant; her older daughter an insecure teenager; her younger daughter a petrified adolescent; my sister an egocentric princess; and I was a starving rebel. The household represented everything I lacked—femininity, nurturance, and emotionality. Rather than huddle with them on the couch watching soaps or sit with them around the kitchen table for hours on end eating, laughing, smoking, and crying, I hid in my room, stayed at my new boyfriend's house, or went to the gym.

At seventeen I had discovered the adrenaline rush and the endorphin boost of a high-speed cardiovascular workout. Aerobics was my new drug of choice. After Kim died, I started starving again. Once my food was back under control and there was nothing else I could cut out or skip, I needed something to intensify what had become the norm. It's at this stage that many anorexics turn to vomiting, laxatives, or diet pills. I turned to what, at a glance, could be misconstrued as an aboveboard fitness practice. Like most anorexics, I turned to compulsive exercising.

Aerobics quickly became an outward manifestation of the madness in my head. Everybody knew about my aerobics obsession because it interfered with everything. I never missed a single Fatburn class, with the same instructor with whom I was obsessed. If I was with friends, I dumped them so I could go to aerobics. If I had an appointment, I canceled it. If I had to study for an exam, I delayed it. In years to come when I would relocate to another city, I would drive an hour each way across an interstate highway just to make it to my Fatburn class. And when I eventually moved overseas and traveled home to visit, I would make international calls to the gym to find out about my Fatburn class, and I would book my plane ticket around it, with enough time to make it to the class after landing.

Even after my life-long awaited eye operation, which my mother didn't want me to have because she said I was too malnourished, I did aerobics. I had waited seventeen years to correct my squint so that I could finally feel normal. I was in the hospital, drugged out, with black stitches coming out of my eyeball. It hurt to open my eye, to look left, right, up, down. It even hurt my eye to bend my body down and run a bath. The doctor's orders were to refrain from any exercise for at least two weeks. I was doing aerobics after two days.

"Please!" my mother begged me. She stood in my bedroom doorway as I sat on the edge of my bed tying my sneakers' laces, pretending I didn't hear her. "You are destroying yourself! You have just had eye surgery, you need to heal, you need to rest, you need to recuperate. Please hear me . . . please."

I stood up and walked toward her. She turned sideways to let me through.

"I'm borrowing your car," I said. "And I am going to the gym!"

Nobody was going to stop me from burning my fat! Aerobics was my binge as well as my purge. I binged on adrenaline and purged the guilt. I felt invincible. Indestructible. In control. The studio doors slid open, and I raced in to grab my regular spot in the front row where I could watch my body in the full-length wall-to-wall mirror. I wore short shorts, a tight tank top, short socks, and white aerobics sneakers. My instructor sauntered in wearing a men's leotard.

"Is everybody ready to pump it tonight?" he yelled. The jam-packed lubricated bodies inside the studio yelled back.

"Yesssssssss!"

"Are we going to work it up to the max?"

"Yessssssssssss!"

"Then go go go! Keep moving it. Push push push. Take it higher and higher . . ."

Hard beats blasted out of four speakers, which was the instructor's cue to pump it up. I pounded the floor, side to side, up and down, the music creeping up my neck. Every second I watched every inch of my body pulse and flex, each muscle contract and tone, and I kept my eye on every curve, angle, and outline of my flesh. My feet hammered the ground, and my arms pulsated in the air. Sweat dripped from the back of my neck down my spine, wetting the floor.

I worshipped the rush I got from pounding my body to the ground. I relied on it to get me through the week. Nothing compared to it. It was the only "pleasure" I allowed myself in all those years because it achieved an end result. It made me thinner and harder and spun me more and more outside of myself. It erased all thoughts and destroyed all feeling.

In the years I overdosed on aerobics, I developed shin splints, which sent a sharp pain surging up my shins every time my feet hit the ground. Friends warned me that so much exercise for so many years on an empty stomach could kill me. My mother screamed at me, begged me, and cried to me to stop the abuse. "But it's just exercise," I'd say. "Exercise is healthy. It's acceptable. It's good for me." I didn't tell her that it was my way to give vent to and grind away at my pain. I didn't tell her that aerobics was my saving grace, the only thing worth living for because it made me feel so good.

In that same year I was a senior in high school majoring in drama, art, and history. Drama was one of the main reasons I chose to attend the convent. Had I not had a creative outlet for my self-expression in those years, I might have imprisoned myself in my own solitary confinement and waited to die. But I wasn't waiting to die. I was fighting to survive. I channeled my creative energy, my anger, my pain, and all that had not yet been annihilated into my acting and art classes. My art portfolio received one of the highest scores in the country. My creative writing was praised by the school's faculty. My name was called at a school assembly, and I went up onstage, in front of the whole school, to receive a trophy in my honor. Or so I'm told. It was the first time in the history of the school that any student had so excelled both in drama and in art. But I would not have remembered any of it had my mom not reminded me of these achievements a few years ago. All that mattered to me at the time was that my food was under control and that my body was in control.

Most of my friends had solid plans to go to universities and get degrees, and I had nothing but my next gym class to look forward to. My mother had longed for the day that I would feel free as a bird, as long as I didn't want to fly too far from her nest. She was slightly older than I was then when she left home and married, and she did not want the same for me. She said university would be stimulating and challenging, but she didn't say I had to go. She wanted to see me get involved in a visual art, like photography, because she thought acting was pretentious. My father, who called himself a student of life, said academic institutions were full of pompous intellectuals who hid behind their books because they were social rejects. He didn't encourage higher academic education and said I should pursue acting because it was my passion. On a trip to London at age twelve, my father prematurely took me to tour top British acting schools, like the Royal Academy of Dramatic Art, which was out of my league, unaffordable and unrealistic seeing as I wasn't living in London. But still, it was an inspirational gesture on his part. A few years later, at age sixteen, on a trip to Israel, my father took me to a filmmaking school to inquire as to whether I could one day apply. They glared at me like I was a fool to ask and told me to come back only once I had gained some life experience.

But despite having spent my last three years in high school

expressing my creativity, I didn't want it anymore. I wasn't conscious of why that was. I wasn't aware that to continue with self-expression would have meant reaching deep inside myself, exploring my inner terrain, and sifting through the pain. Instead, I said that acting was indulgent and self-centered and art was boring because it was something at which I was naturally talented. The truth was that I didn't want to be deep or challenged. My life felt complicated enough as it was. I wanted to do shallow, banal things because I was desperate to find simplicity and ease.

"The world is your oyster," my mother said to me on the day I finished high school. But what does a girl do with freedom at seventeen? I'll tell you what I did: nothing. I lay on the couch in the living room every day for three weeks, staring into space, my head like a boulder too heavy to lift, my body a brick, with my limbs cemented into the couch. One day, my mother walked past me, holding a paintbrush in one hand and clenching another paintbrush between her teeth. She smeared her paint-stained hands on her overalls, replaced the paintbrush in her mouth with a cigarette, lit it, and rolled her eyes at me.

"Stop moping," she said as she turned around, choking me with her smoke.

But I wasn't moping. I was scared. I was lost. I was depressed. I had no idea who I was supposed to be in the big wide world. I had no idea who I was, let alone what I wanted to do with my life. *If being me is the root of my pain,* I thought, *then I will have to deny who I am in every single way. I will deny my roots, deny my creativity, and deny my mother. But first,* I thought, *I will lie here on this couch and wish that I had the energy to get up and drag my body to the garden to bury my head in the smoke of my mother's stolen cigarettes.*

Many years later, I would meet a girl at my yoga studio. She was eighteen, and I was twenty-something. We took the same classes and greeted each other with hellos and goodbyes, hugs and kisses. One day she sauntered into class glowing. She wore her hair up in a bright orange hair wrap, and she sat on the floor, her back upright, her legs crossed in lotus pose, and her arms outstretched with her palms turned up to the sky. I approached her after class. I wanted to know her secret. Was she in love? Pregnant?

"I just graduated from high school," she told me. "It's so amazing that now I get to practice yoga every day and go for walks on the beach every morning and surf the waves every afternoon. I have all the time in the world to do absolutely everything I love: draw, paint, write poetry. I mean, how awesome is life? I've started saving up to backpack around the world next year . . ."

I thought back to the weeks following my high school graduation. After lying immobile and catatonic on the couch day in and day out, I tore out an ad I had found in the classifieds. A beauty salon was hiring manicurists to do false nails. I showed it to my mother and told her I wanted to try it. She laughed and told me to get a life. My friend Leah was going to be doing an aerobics instructor's course, so I applied with her, and we practiced aerobics twice a day for a couple of months. But I didn't pass the theory exam, so I didn't qualify. My friend Cindy signed up for a typing course, and I decided to do that with her. I dressed up in mismatched skirts and jackets pretending to be mature, secretary-like. I was angry that I had too many choices and no direction. I wanted guidance, but I didn't know what to call it at the time. When faced with a world of opportunity, all I wanted to do was escape.

Many years later I would meet the same girl at my yoga studio again. She had returned from her global escapade, and she looked withdrawn.

"What's wrong?" I asked. "I've never seen you look so down before."

"Oh, it's nothing serious," she answered. "It's just a feeling inside."

I wished I could have said the same for myself all those years.

It's just a feeling inside.

Chapter Eight

HEARTBREAK

Toward the end of high school, my father decided to relocate to Israel once more, this time on his own, to start his life over again. Months later, when he suggested I come live with him, he promised me a car, a stereo, and a TV. I accepted. I know exactly what I was thinking when I decided to move there six months after graduation. I was thinking that this was my opportunity to reclaim the happiness that I had been forced to leave behind in Israel at age seven and that finally, now that I was grown up, my father would love me and talk to me. But almost as soon as I arrived, our relationship teetered on the edge of ruin. He had no time for what he called my "teenage crap," for my slut clothes, my arrogant boyfriend, and my narcissistic desires. We had not lived together for longer than one consecutive week in ten years. He had no idea how to handle a teenager far away from her home, her roots, trying to push her way into a hardened society. And he absolutely did not know how to save a teenager from struggling with herself.

My dad picked me up from the airport the day I arrived. I wore tight hipster jeans and a short spaghetti-strap top that exposed my lean belly. I pushed a trolley load of two bags the size of treasure chests through the sliding doors and looked for his face in the crowd. I spotted him on his phone, speaking loud and pacing up and down. I walked up to him, and he covered the mouthpiece and held his pointing finger to my face as if to say, *Give me a minute, I'm on the phone, this is very important.*

I waited.

"What shit are you wearing?" he said, closing his phone. He hugged me tentatively. "Pull your pants up. Your jeans are so fucking low that everyone can see your pubic hair."

I swallowed.

"And why have you lost so much weight, again?" he said. "I told you, it doesn't suit you."

He took a step back to look at me, shook his head from side to side, and threw his arms in the air as if to say, *I give up.*

Instead he said, "I don't know who is worse, you or your mother!"

The first thing I noticed was his gold watch and his new shoes. He looked expensive. And smelled expensive. He wore an ironed checked collared shirt and fitted jeans, both designer labels.

"I'll buy you new clothes because you can't walk around looking like a leftover," he said.

I said nothing. I felt heat rise in my chest and my throat close and my stomach squeeze. I held my breath until I couldn't hold it in any longer. He put his arm around me and pushed the trolley out of the airport terminal.

"Wait till you see my new car," he said. "You won't believe your eyes."

Growing up, my father was absent even when he was around.

"I've got nothing in common with kids. I'll be able to talk

to you when you are more grown up," he said to my sister and me all throughout our childhood. So we waited. We waited for him to look up from his piles of weekend newspapers. We waited for the end of the game blaring on TV. We waited for him to get off the phone that was glued to his ear while he conducted his business deals. And we waited for the news on the hour every hour to end before asking a question or sharing our own news.

After my parents' divorce, my father, who at that point had no money, moved from a crummy granny cottage to a dinky flat in a run-down building. Every abode he ever lived in felt like a corporate office with a bed. The only things in the kitchen cupboard were packets of instant mashed potatoes. Add hot water and stir. My sister and I played Monopoly with him just to be close to him. We choreographed dances to his music—The Best of George Benson—just so he would watch. And every Saturday night when he took us to skate, we wished he would hold our hands on the ice. But my dad always had something better to do, something more important, a business deal to close, a business partner to call, money to make, people to see, and places to go. I spent more time sitting in the back of his luxury cars (no matter how little money he made, he always had a luxury car) staring at the back of his head than I did speaking to him. If I hadn't had my sister by my side as my best friend and playmate, I might have disappeared into the loneliness.

He took us to video stores to get take-away entertainment. He left us to choose. We lay on blankets behind the couch in our man-made movie house. My dad pressed play on the video machine and left the room. We watched teenagers in college scrambling for sex and partying and driving drunk. All the girls had big breasts and small voices, and all the boys had six-pack abs and only one thing on their minds. The nerds had nothing. We did not know that the number twenty-one on a video's back cover was an age restriction, and my father never checked it. I remember one scene with a girl sitting on the floor with her legs spread in the splits. She wore a leotard and made sex noises into the phone. We told my mother what we saw, and she called my dad.

"What were you thinking? They are children!" she yelled.

"Calm down! It's not like they were watching blue movies!" my dad said.

I know that my father would have rather died than end up living like a student again. My mother had my sister and me and her passion for her art and the house of her dreams. My father had a failed marriage, the loss of his children, and the unfulfilled dream of a happy family. He took the divorce worse than my mother because he had to start over alone and redefine his role outside of our family. But I took it worse than either of them. More than anything else in the whole world, I wanted my father's love, and eventually I would do almost anything to get it.

A couple of years later, when I was eleven, he moved to a house with a lush atrium, a banana tree that blew in the wind, and a swimming pool that sparkled under the African sun. It was in a family-oriented neighborhood next to a park that we never went to because he was busy with his carpet business. His business was picking up, and he had less and less time for us. He shouted swear words into the phone while we lay around on piles of Persian carpets, blocking our ears and jumping from one pile to the next pretending they were giant stepping stones in a stream. He took us everywhere he went—to look at show houses, to make bank deposits, to close business deals, to buy bigger and better electronic systems and upgrade to the latest technology. My mother was pleased for him that he finally lived in a beautiful home and that he could work in a spacious office next to the pool. My sister and I visited on weekends, reluctantly. We visited him because he was our father, and each time we hoped it would be different. But every weekend was the same, year after year. From the moment we arrived at his house he had the TV on at full volume with sports commentators barking at a game of rugby or soccer or cricket. He refused to turn it off or turn the volume down and told us that "just being in the same room is enough" and "we don't need to talk to feel like we are spending time together." He pointed to piles of old newspapers and magazines and said, "Entertain yourselves."

I remember occupying myself for hours on end with my own head games. I sat next to him on the couch pining for his attention, hoping he would put his arm around me or tell me I could rest my head on his chest. Instead, I sat tight and paged through one of his outdated tabloid magazines, which he bought so he could do the crossword puzzles. I paged through them like they were photo albums of precious memories. I pretended that each person on each page was someone from my class, and I made up stories in my head and tried to blot out the noise of the TV in the background. To this day I would rather have the reverberation of dozens of glass bottles breaking in my ears than those sports commentators' voices.

My dad bought us a red metal bunk bed, and whenever we arrived to spend the weekend at his house, the beds were just as we had left them because nobody ever went into the room. The duvets smelled dusty and felt scratchy and our pillows were stuffed with synthetics. At night when we were tucked in bed lying still in corpse pose, my dad came to kiss us goodnight. I told him I was cold. He tucked the duvet tighter around my body and said that soon enough I would forget about it.

We couldn't have settled down in his houses even if we had wanted to because in a matter of months he would up and leave for something bigger, something better. His houses were as transient as his girlfriends, who he flicked through like they were boring TV channels. Each one was more beautiful than the last, he said. He bought them expensive gifts and took them on lavish business trips overseas. My mother says that his girlfriends wore the child-support money owed to her around their necks and wrists.

"Don't you think she is stunning?" my dad asked me about each girlfriend. "Why don't you dress like that? Why don't you want me to buy you shoes like that? Why do always look like such a leftover? You've got no style."

I was eleven. All I wanted was for him to call me beautiful, just once, so I would know I was worthy in his eyes. But I was never pretty enough, clever enough, or perfect enough for him. I was never like one of his girlfriends.

Other than his girlfriends and clients, there was no one around; there were no dinners or parties or music except when he was in a romantic mood and listened to The Best of George Benson or *Phantom of the Opera*. The feeling in his house was that same empty creepy feeling I felt in my belly over the years, which later would define my whole world. It was the feeling of a house that wasn't lived in. A house that wasn't a home. His houses were like temporary motel rooms or office cubicles. Where my mother had lush land and abundant undergrowth, my father had a few dying orchids planted in dried-out pots because nobody ever watered them.

His houses were littered with broken gadgets and wires, plugs and pens, men's deodorant and cologne, tabloid magazines, piles of newspapers, and ultra-sweet air freshener. His shelves were lined with crystal wine glasses, and his living room had bronze sculptures balancing on glass pedestals. "Don't touch! You'll break it! Leave it alone! Be careful!" he yelled. And the more money he made, the more he spent on things that we children could break. His appliances got bigger and slimmer, his fast cars were replaced with faster cars, and his crockery was upgraded to more expensive top-of-the-line designs. And the more he upgraded his assets, the more he downgraded me. I was the inappropriately dressed, nagging child who walked in front of the TV, opened the car door without looking, touched what I wasn't supposed to, and asked the wrong questions, all of which were stupid.

As my sister and I got older, we stopped going to his houses. Instead, he collected us from my mom and took us out for dinner, which was the only time he was able to concentrate because there were no technological distractions. But as soon as the conversation was over and we had covered the generic subjects, like how we did on our exams, how high we scored, how our friendships were going at school, and how our mom was doing with her art, there was nothing more to say. Our relationship faded like an old stain on clothing that you don't even want to wear anymore.

My father never had parents on whom to model his parenting style. His father had abandoned the family early on, and his mother had then sent my father, and his older brother, to an orphanage at the age of two. His mother, who had recently immigrated to Israel from Austria, had remarried and had another child, and her new husband refused to support my father and his brother so they remained at the orphanage while her third child lived with her at home. As a teenager, my father continued his studies at a boarding school where he integrated well. At age eighteen, he was conscripted into the Israel Defense Force and served his time in the paratroopers unit. He learned to fight, to survive, to be hard and resilient. As a child I had taken all his hardness personally, and by the time I turned eighteen, I was ready to give it back.

Growing up, that was just about as much as I knew about him. I heard the same stories again and again, but I wanted to know more. I wanted to know where he came from and who he was, how he grew up and what he was like in those years. I wanted to get to know his mother and sleep in her house, which he had visited only on vacations. This man was my father, an enigma, and I wanted so much to piece together his life so that I could begin to piece together my other roots. That was why I decided to move to Israel after high school—to reclaim my happiness and to understand my father so that I could better understand myself. I hoped that at the same time he would finally love me the way I wanted to be loved.

The day I arrived at the Israeli airport at age eighteen, he drove me to his apartment, which was in one of the wealthiest neighborhoods in Tel Aviv. His open-plan dining-room-cum-living-area had a varnished oval wood dining table and elegant chairs with silk cushions, a massive flat-screen TV, and a velvet chaise to lounge on. In the corner was a sofa that he had upholstered in imported designer material and a glass-topped coffee table with fragile, expensive ornaments that belonged in a glass case in a museum. A black leather recliner chair was in another corner on a small Persian rug beside a bookshelf packed with art and antique collectors' books. He showed me to my room. It had a single bed, an empty TV stand, and a pine dresser that was missing a few drawer handles.

Later, he introduced me to his Hungarian girlfriend. "She is not like the others," he told me. "This one is special. The love of my life." She was petite, with soft skin as if from a soap advertisement. She had jade eyes that kept you at a distance and a pinched nose that made her nostrils look like slits. She wore the right shoes—white moccasins with neat tassels. Her thin ankles, with perfect Vs at her anklebones, stuck out under her cream chinos. Her pale blue ironed shirt was buttoned up to just below her neck, and she wore a delicate gold necklace like a strand of saffron with a diamond in the middle. She looked like the pampered wife of a wealthy man, sailing in the Caribbean on a yacht. She put her soft moisturized hand out to greet me, and I almost gave a curtsy in response. *If this is my father's idea of perfection*, I thought, *then I have a hell of a long way to go.* I tucked my hands, with my bitten fingernails, into my torn jean pockets and asked her if I could smoke one of her ultra-slim menthol cigarettes. A puppy bounded out of the kitchen yelping, and my father shouted at her to shut up. She was a purebred Weimaraner with fur as soft as her new mother's skin. "This is our baby," his girlfriend told me. Months later, this woman would give my father an ultimatum. She said she could not live with a teenager. He would have to choose. Eventually her ultimatum would backfire on her.

One night, my father hosted one of his once-in-a-blue-moon dinner parties. I was smoking unfiltered cigarettes in my room and listening to Phil Collins's "Against All Odds" on my small stereo. I strolled out in my jean shorts and tank top to get a drink of water from the kitchen. The adults were drinking red wine, and I asked my dad if I could have some. He didn't hear me, so I grabbed an upside-down crystal glass off the table. "Not that one," he shouted. "You'll break it!" *Like you break me*, I thought. I put the crystal glass down slowly and walked into the kitchen, to get myself a regular glass, swearing under my breath. The dog was chewing on a piece of black lace.

"That's mine," I yelled, yanking it out her mouth. The Weimaraner scampered under the coffee table with her amputated tail between her legs. I threw the piece of wet tattered lace at my father's feet, stormed off to my bedroom, locked the door behind me, and lit up a cigarette.

Later that night, I shouted at him, "You don't give a shit that your dog ate my G-string!"

He burst out laughing uncontrollably and turned to walk away.

"Stop laughing, Daddy! It's not funny! That was mine! Why should I respect your things if you don't respect me?"

A year later, I would move with him to another suburb just outside of Tel Aviv into a two-story house with a garden and four bedrooms. He said he wanted something bigger. And better. I chose a room that had red wall-to-wall carpeting the color of a rose as it starts to wilt. Three carpeted steps led up to a raised level with a single mattress on it. The sliding cupboard doors were mirrored from floor to ceiling, and the windows had thick dark wood blinds. I chose the red room because at first it felt regal, like a palace with a red carpet leading up to it, but when the blinds were shut, it turned into a dungeon where I kept the princess in me captive.

Looking back at that time I realize that I used smoking, drinking, and casual sex to escape my self-imposed captivity. One outlet for my pent-up rage that got exacerbated in Israel was stealing. I continued to steal clothing that I didn't need, or really want, from stores. Only once did I get caught by a store owner who threatened to call my father unless I paid him triple what the item was worth, which I did using my father's money for groceries. Since I was now handling a lot of money waiting tables, for the first time in Israel, I started pocketing cash from customer's paid bills and landed up taking home ten times the amount that I would have earned in tips alone. I didn't do anything with the money. Instead, just knowing I got away with it, made me feel powerful and invincible.

The day after my nineteenth birthday, which I had spent alone and melancholic in the house after my father, before going out for the night, had ordered me a pizza as a birthday present—which I didn't eat—I was asleep in my red dungeon when he charged into my room and let out a roar.

"Get up! It's eight in the morning! Why are you still sleeping?"

My eyes flew open, and my heart beat faster. "But it's Saturday!" I snapped back.

"You are fucking lazy, and this room is a pigsty! Get out of bed and make the most of your day. Pick up all the shit off the floor; your clothes are everywhere."

He pointed to a glass ashtray next to my bed overflowing with cigarettes stubs.

"And empty out that ashtray right now! It's disgusting." He turned around and left the door wide open. I heard his voice trailing behind him as he stomped downstairs: "Like a fucking cockroach . . ."

I peeled the sheet off me, like you would while identifying a body in a morgue, and plunked my feet on the steps. I bent over and folded my arms over my knees, and my head fell onto my arms. I looked at the mound of stale cigarette butts. *What's the big deal?* I thought. *This is my room, not his. He has no right to charge in here and make demands on me.* I was wearing a short, tight spaghetti-strap top and hot pants. I got up and picked up the glass ashtray, still tipsy from being half asleep. I yawned my way downstairs, holding onto the rail with one hand and clasping the ashtray in the other. I zombie-walked to the kitchen. My father stood at the sink, wearing yellow rubber gloves, washing the dishes. I dumped the cigarette butts into the trashcan next to him.

"What the fuck are you doing?" he yelled. "Don't be stupid! Can't you see there is no plastic bag inside? Why don't you open your eyes and look! You are fucking selfish, do you know that? You have no respect!"

His rubber-gloved hand splashed into the water like a bird that was shot out of the sky. The dishwater dripped wet on his sleeve, and he ripped off the gloves.

"I didn't fucking see it! I was half asleep. I hadn't even opened my eyes yet, and you stormed into my bedroom giving me orders!" I yelled, backing away.

"The problem is that you are fucking lazy and you live in a pigsty!" he screamed.

I pressed my palm onto the marble kitchen counter and dug my heels into the marble tiled floor. "So what? It is none of your fucking business, Daddy! It's my—"

"It is my house! Do you understand me? You are living under my roof, and you will do what I say! Go back there and clean up that mess in your room and put on some clothes! You can't walk around here like a slut!"

He screamed so hard I thought he would start foaming soap suds from his mouth.

"I am not a fucking slut!" I yelled, my voice screeching like tires on a wet road. "Get off my back and leave me alone, Daddy! Stop screaming at me all the fucking time! Since when do you think you can come into my life and tell me what to do?"

"The problem is that you have no fucking respect—for any of my things!" he yelled.

"NO! The problem is that you have no fucking respect for me!"

He grabbed the wet dish sponge out of the dirty water and threw it at my face. "Fuck you!" he yelled.

"No! Fuck YOU!" I yelled back, wiping the water off my face.

His arm swung toward me, and I felt a sharp sting on my cheek. I lost my balance and fell to the ground screaming. He climbed onto me to hold down my thrashing arms.

"That's right!" I screamed. "Fucking hit me!" I was an animal that would fight until its death. But suddenly he got up and took a few steps back. The room fell silent, and I realized I stopped screaming. I picked myself up off the floor and backed away caressing my cheek.

"I hope you are sorry," I said, softly choking on my words. "I hope you are very, very sorry . . ."

I ran upstairs and slammed my bedroom door behind me and bent over, heaving like I had sprinted in a race. I grabbed a pair of jeans off the floor and threw on a T-shirt and pulled sneakers onto my bare feet. I shoved the mirrored cupboard door to the side and fumbled around on the top shelf for a duffle bag, into which I stuffed more clothes. Miniature bottles of alcohol that I'd stolen from airplanes were lined up neatly on a shelf. I downed vodka and tequila and rum and chucked more bottles into the bag, zipped it up, flung it over my shoulder, and stormed out.

I walked around the house looking for my father and found him in the basement organizing his artworks swathed in bubble wrap and carefully stacked against the walls. Tears streamed down my hot face, and sweat soaked my armpits. I put my chest forward like a pigeon and clenched my jaw and stared him down. He was kneeling down on one of his expensive Persian rugs wrapping in bubble wrap a bronze sculpture, a figure of a woman in a wispy dress. He pressed his elbow on his knee when he saw me and stood up slowly.

"I came here to tell you," I said through my heaving breaths, "that I am leaving, and I am never coming back."

I felt myself go weak at the knees and my gut sucking in like a punctured ball.

"I want you to know that I will never forgive you," I gasped. "You will die a lonely old man. You will die alone, and nobody will come to your funeral. Nobody."

The air in the room was so dense that I felt I might stop breathing. My father stood dead still without blinking. In his hand he held a piece of bubble wrap with pieces of ripped masking tape stuck to the ends. I turned around and walked away and left him standing there, surrounded by all his protected precious pieces.

I walked for hours through the suburbs, across fields, over a bridge, and along a highway with the desert sun burning my neck red. I walked for hours until I reached the city center of Tel Aviv, where I checked myself in to a tourist hostel for the night. I felt untouchable. Nobody could hurt me. I had survived.

I don't remember how I got back to my father's house the following day, but I knew I had nowhere else to go. I found him slumped on the couch staring at a blank black TV screen. His glazed eyes were wet. He looked broken. I felt sorry for him. I saw my father in pain. For the first time ever, he looked vulnerable. He spoke in a whisper and said he was sorry. I knew he meant it. He begged me to stay and to give it another chance. He promised me that things would get better.

I wanted so much to believe him.

But things only got worse, and a few months later we had another huge fight, this time over the telephone, after he asked to borrow my car as his was getting repaired and I said no, because I needed it.

"You are not my daughter," he said. "I disown you." After he slammed the phone down on me, I felt the blood drain out of my body, and my hands started shaking and I went weak at the knees. I stood dead still, holding the telephone receiver against my aching, racing heart, repeating to myself the most painful sentence I had ever heard: *You are not my daughter; I disown you.* With those few words, my father had affirmed my deeply held belief that I wasn't worthy. I wasn't good enough. I wasn't lovable. And I accepted it. I believed it. I owned it.

Chapter Nine

LIGHTNING AT SUNSET

One month before leaving for Israel, just before my eighteenth birthday, my twenty-seven-year-old aerobics instructor approached me after class. As casually as though he were asking the time, he said, "Do you want to have sex?" When I heard myself say yes, it affirmed my belief that to be desired by a man meant one thing only: that I was worthy.

In Israel, anonymous and alone in a new country, I needed all the self-worth I could get. I was a new immigrant wanting desperately to fit in to Israeli society, and an insecure teenager wanting even more to be wanted. In my first week there, I exchanged numbers with some guy I met in a shopping mall at a shoe store. A few days later we had sex on a beach, and he never called me again. Even though I was not particularly interested in him—I can't even remember what he looked like—I did not think it was a one-night stand. I called his house every day for weeks and begged his siblings to get him to come to the phone, hoping that maybe he was not as cruel and cold-hearted like I was beginning to think he might be. Maybe he was just a young guy who got what he wanted and thought I had too. But I didn't know what I really wanted from him. I just knew that I did not want the pain of feeling rejected.

Years later I would learn to empathize with the girl that I was. Even if she didn't know what she wanted, she wasn't looking for what she got. It would take a lot of therapy to learn that a boy's hugs and kisses would not soothe my deepest of pains. But in the meantime, I wore the sweatshirt he lent me that night, every day for months, as though it would offer me the comfort, the warmth that I was searching for by going with him in the first place.

In Israel I ate more than I was eating before. Maybe it was the novelty of a new culture, the freedom of being away from my mother's watchful eye, or the feeling that I was getting special treatment from my father when he prepared food for me. I found a job waiting tables at a beachfront restaurant-cum-bar. The manager was a pot-bellied middle-aged man who reeked of cologne. He offered to give me a ride home after work one night. He parked outside my father's apartment. I thanked him, and he took the liberty of grabbing me by the back of my neck like you would a cat, pulling my face toward his, and thrusting his slimy tongue down my throat. I pulled away and ran upstairs to spit. I continued to work there for months but never accepted another ride from him.

At the same restaurant I met a lovely guy, a bartender, who treated me with respect and care, but I was so suspicious of his kindness that after hanging out many times as close friends, when he took me to his place and shared with me that he wanted to make love to me, I was so freaked out that I got up and left. It was like my body just didn't recognize the loving kindness he was sending my way so it was treated like a foreign invader. To let love in would have required me to soften and allow myself to feel my feelings, and that felt way more scary at the time than letting horny, abusive guys have their way with me.

On Saturday mornings, a small group of men in their forties

and fifties used the beach in front of the restaurant to set up and
ride their Jet Skis. I had always wanted to cruise the seas. After
work one Saturday, I asked one of them for a ride. He told me
to come back the next week in my bikini. I did. He told me to
sit in front, and he got on behind me and wrapped his arms
around my waist and we shot off. When we were far from land,
he slid his hand down and crept his fingers under my bikini bottom. I didn't think to stop him. The Jet Ski cruised onto a deserted beach far from land, and we climbed off. I sat away from
him on the beach, frozen. I told him I wanted to go back. I
don't remember if anything else happened, but he dumped me
back on land, and I never went on another Jet Ski. I didn't tell
anybody about this until years later in therapy—not because I
was ashamed, but because I wasn't sure that what he did was
wrong.

Later, I met a soldier whose job it was to wash dishes in the
army. He told me he did karate, and I thought we found common
ground because I had done karate as a kid. We went to a bar one
night and got drunk, and I went home with him. I remember
that he heaved his oafish body on top of me and I squirmed
around underneath his weight and mumbled something about
how I was trying to say no to sex, wanting to respect myself. A
friend had told me that if I just knew who I was, then nobody
could take that away from me because it was worth everything. I
thought of that friend as my savior. But a savior is useless when
you can't save yourself. The next morning, I woke up next to
this stranger in bed, nauseous from the hangover and the familiar,
sick mix of failure and shame. I was naked except for my G-
string. I hugged my legs to my chest and wrapped my arms
around my shins and quietly rocked myself to and fro. *Why
couldn't you just say no?* I thought. *Why did you have to fail in the
simple task you set for yourself of saying no?* I left his house that

day and never spoke to him again. I cried on the few occasions that something reminded me of him, although I had no real understanding of why.

Months later I picked up a guy in a club whose name in Hebrew means *lightning*. I was nineteen, he was twenty-nine, and to me he represented Man—gorgeous, solid, distant. He was a deep-sea diver who fixed washing machines for a living and juggled with devil sticks and knives in his free time. I wrote in my diary that he scared me, that he looked evil and manipulative and abusive. I wrote, *Why do I choose men with evil eyes?*

The first time I went home with him, I discovered that he also liked to draw, that we had the same taste in music, and that we used the same soap. I thought these extraneous details defined him, which in my mind meant he was right for me, good for me. He told me he thought I was cute and lovable. I did not believe him. I told him he had the face of a killer and the hands of a spider. He kept saying, "You poor thing, what have they done to you?" I wanted him to hold me and protect me. He wanted me to strip down to my G-string and called me a party pooper when I refused. After a few dates, he got bored with my mistrust and paranoia. He said he had fantasized about me but that I turned out to be a nice, normal girl. He said I needed a long time to recuperate.

"Recuperate from what?" I asked.

"From life," he said. He saw my fear but still did not understand why I refused to have sex with him after he said, "I want to fuck you till you bleed."

I wrote in my diary at the time how much I hated men, how much they had hurt me. But I was young and vulnerable, and I had no comprehension of consequence, no understanding of lust not being love. A part of me honestly believed, in all my gullibility that I would live happily ever after with some guy I picked up in a shoe store. Or that a gorgeous man who told me he wanted to fuck me till I bled was actually capable of loving me with real kindness. Or that having one trivial thing in common with some stranger meant everlasting love.

In between these flings, I met a guy, a fellow waiter at the beach bar, who told me months into our relationship that the only reason he had sex with me in the first place was that he was dared to by the bartender I had already slept with. He won the dare and more. After one week of dating, I was madly in love with him. We spent every minute together. He told me he loved me. I said the same. He dared me to drive with him to a beach resort in the Sinai desert, and I accepted. He had a scooter, and my father had bought me a beat-up Volkswagen Beetle that looked bright and orange but was low on life. He said he was up for adventure but what he had really wanted was a ride.

A few weeks later, we were on the road to the desert. My Beetle engine puttered and choked for a few miles until it came to a standstill and blew up. He was driving. He slammed the steering wheel with his fists and kicked open the door. I felt something sticky between my legs. I got up and pointed at the blood-stained seat. I had forgotten it was that time of the month again. "Thanks! Now we can't even have sex!" he yelled. He slammed his hands on the car roof and kicked the tire with his foot and blamed me for ruining his vacation.

I soaked up guilt as though it were nourishment. Any sane person would have left him standing on the side of the road and run as fast and as far as possible. But I hitched us a ride by showing off my tight denim shorts and called my father once we got to the Egyptian border. He told me to come home. I ranted and begged and got him to tow the car back to Tel Aviv. We crossed the border into Egypt. My boyfriend flashed his electric smile and pulled me toward him for a hard tongue kiss. That was how I allowed my nineteen-year-old boyfriend to treat me. In line with how I treated myself. Only when it came from him, I called it love.

Months later we were drinking beers at an outdoor club on the beach. I wore skin-tight pants and a glittering pale blue halter top that showed off my belly-ringed, suntanned stomach. We were locked in a clawed embrace, our eyes sucked each other in, and our hands crawled all over each other's bodies. We downed our beers and smoked our cigarettes. Then he told me to go to the bar and order another round. The black sea crashed in the background, and the boom of the Trance party gained speed. I ordered two more beers and returned to find him where I left him, with his slick smile and gleaming brown eyes. But his neck was taut and his hands were in fists.

"I saw how you looked at him," he snapped.

"Who?"

"You know who. Your eyes were all over him at the bar." His smile narrowed, and his jaw locked. I trembled and felt a knot in my gut. I had no idea who he was even talking about. I didn't notice any guys at the bar. I set the beers down on the wooden slat that he leaned against. It was the one thing that separated us from the dark abyss of salty water. He grabbed my wrist and pulled me away from the wood slats and into the pulsing crowd. "We are leaving!" he said as he stormed out and pulled me along like I was at the end of his chain. My car was parked in a packed lot. It stood out in the night because of its bright orange color—ironically, the color of joy. I heard my father's voice in my head: *Leave him! He is a piece of shit! He is nothing. Tell him to fuck off.*

But I love him. I love him. I will do anything for him. Anything.

As we walked toward my car, three skinny guys in tight

jeans with heavy gold chains around their necks and their hair gelled up in Mohawks strolled past us. One of the guys dangled a cigarette out of his mouth, and his wrist was clad with fake silver chains. He stank of cologne. He turned around and grabbed me by the back of my pants, and I stumbled. Then he swiped his hand under my groin from front to back and ran off with his friends laughing. They gave one another high fives that sounded like bombs. I glanced at my boyfriend, expecting him to do something. Instead, he warned me not to mess with "guys like that" and kept walking until I caught up with him.

My boyfriend and I stood on either side of my car as he spat out his accusations about the guy at the bar like darts. One after another, I dodged them or caught them until I could take no more. I had not eaten anything all day (although I was going through a stage of eating more than usual) and was rushing on cigarettes and alcohol. The anger in me was so big that my whole body convulsed and my fingers spread like a cat's paws.

I want to rip your throat open. I want to tear your body apart. I want to smash your head into this car.

The car acted as a metal barricade that sliced the space between us. He yelled. I yelled louder. He swore. I swore dirty. Suddenly I stopped screaming, and there was a quiet so strong I could not even hear myself breathe. I felt a stinging on my arm. I was gripping my car key in one hand. I looked down at my peachy forearm, at where it was stinging. There were lines of bright red bloody gashes carved into my skin. Like my skin had been plowed. There was my blood on the car key. I did not know at the time that there was a name for what I had discovered. I did not know that I would come to depend on cutting many more times over the years to pacify my uncontrollable wrath. I just knew it did something. It killed the feelings.

A couple of months later, my boyfriend and I lay cuddled up

in each other's arms all day on a crowded beach. His arms were wrapped around me as the sea sparkled gently and the bright light began to fade. Suddenly he jumped up and said he wanted to leave. I said I wanted to stay and watch the sunset. He grabbed my car keys. I tugged at his arm, and he pulled away and stormed off.

"Where are you going?" I yelled after him. "Give me back my keys!"

I jumped up and chased after him. He broke into a sprint. I yelled after him, "Give them back!"

People turned to stare, and the sun shot me its rays. I moved in slow motion. I caught up with him and grabbed him by the arm. He swung around and whacked me across the face. I heard a clap and fell to my knees in the sand. He ran off. People ran up to me. Someone put his hand on my head and asked, "Is that your boyfriend?"

I nodded yes. "Don't ever let anyone treat you that way!" I looked up at the glaring sun. Coincidentally, the man who had spoken was the guy that I had picked up in the shoe store and had never heard from again. I still wore his sweatshirt at night. We acknowledged each other casually with "Oh, it's you," or some variation of recognition that fitted the awkwardness of the encounter. He lifted me to my feet and gave me a warm sideways hug like a big brother. I thanked him and walked back to where I had left my towel and packed up our things. The sun was a stunning stinging strip of scarlet pink, and then it was gone. I walked across the beach, people turned to stare, and I found my boyfriend sitting on a rock gazing at the horizon. He got up. Neither of us said a word. We walked side by side to my car. I handed him the keys that he had dropped in the sand when he hit me. He grabbed them, climbed into the driver's seat, and lit a cigarette. I got into the passenger's seat, sat dead still, and stared out my rolled-down window. As we drove off, I let the hot wind suck me away, unaware that the one thing I had left behind on the beach that day was my dignity.

Chapter Ten

GRAPES AND POPCORN

I had been living in Israel for all of three months when I received a letter in the mail informing me that I was to be conscripted into the Israeli army. I thought it was a joke. It wasn't. Because I had lived there as a child, I was classified as a "returning minor." I had an Israeli father and Israeli citizenship, and I had arrived at exactly the right age for service. I would not be exempt from duty. I was told that I had two months to decide whether to spend the next twenty-one months in the Israel Defense Force. If I chose not to serve, I would be deported. And I would then only be allowed to visit Israel as a tourist for three weeks a year until the age of twenty-two.

When you are eighteen, four years seems like a lifetime away. When you are eighteen and sick in the head, a decision of this magnitude is too overwhelming to contemplate rationally. I was consumed by it. I spent hours on the phone mulling it over with my mother in South Africa, who thought the idea was ludicrous. "Are you mad? What do you need this for in your life? Come home to where you can get the love and support you need." My father, on the other hand, said, "It will do you good. You will start to understand what it means to be disciplined, and it will give you a sense of responsibility and some rules. Do it!"

Soon after the call-up, my father left to go on a short business trip overseas. The day he left, I stopped eating. Completely. I felt proud of my abstinence, my resistance, my willpower. To me it meant that I was coping. I was able to control the situation. I didn't understand that because I was in a crisis, I was turning away from food completely. I had no idea that it was actually a desperate attempt to give myself what I needed. I needed some guideline so that I would know how to go about making such a huge decision. When my mother called and asked me how I was doing, I said I was fine. Never mind lonely, scared, starving, petrified, sick, and insane . . . never mind all of that, I was fine—and I believed it.

On the fifth day of my tacit hunger strike (except for two fruits), a couple of friends from South Africa arrived in Israel, and I went to meet them at a youth hostel in Tel Aviv. It was the first time I had left the apartment in five days. I walked through town awake in a dream. Everyone around me played merry-go-round parts in my matinee. Nothing was real. I found Cindy and Angelique in their dorm, slouching on a bunk bed with a couple of dreadlocked suntanned guys wearing shark-tooth-pendant necklaces and surfer shorts. I envied my friends' casual independence, their freedom from parental influences, mixing with backpackers from around the globe. But the decadence and hedonism scared me; running wild in the world with nothing but a backpack and a free spirit made me feel small and vulnerable. I felt far safer alone in my father's apartment watching numbing TV and eating a total of two ripe peaches in five days than hanging out with stoned revelers on a soul mission to let go and find freedom.

Cindy and Angelique got off the bed to hug me. They had braided hair and wore flowing hippie skirts in bright happy col-

ors, beaded necklaces, leather sandals, and toe rings. I was
dressed from head to toe in black. They took me to a doughnut
shop and bought one with chocolate icing cascading over the
sides and another lavishly decorated with hundreds of colored
sprinkles. When it came my turn to order, I used my same old
lame excuse: "I'm not hungry."

"We're going to Egypt next week. Wanna come? We're
taking a dhow down the Nile River. It's gonna be amazing.
Please come!" They wanted me to join them. I wanted to be able
to feel excited, but all I felt was fear. I had a secret life to lead
that needed my undivided attention. Besides, what would they
say if they saw that I ate nothing? They would tell my mother.
They would expose my secret, which was all I felt I owned.
There was no way I could risk it. So I told them I couldn't go. I
had a huge decision to make regarding the army. I needed time
alone to think. And the world needed to stand still for me to do
that.

That night, my father returned. His girlfriend cooked pasta.
I ate. I was starving.

For ten years I had dreamed of being an Israeli. I dreamed of the
freedom I had when I lived there as a child, the feeling of being
accepted and belonging. I longed to understand my father's
roots, to be able to finally relate to his stories of his time in the
army and to bond with him like I could only do if I knew where
he came from. I wanted to know the other side of me, the side
that was not my mother.

I had been in Israel less than six months when I began my
service in the Israel Defense Force. I was eighteen and a soldier.
There would be nothing but rules and regulations and structure
and boundaries and punishment for breaking the rules. Sadly, it

was exactly what I needed. In the army there would be no room for creativity, no opportunity to express my individuality, no room to be me. It was perfect.

I got on a bus loaded with young recruits from all over the country and headed off for three weeks of basic training. We trained all day and slept only four hours a night; the rest of the time we took turns standing outside in the cold guarding the dorm room. We got up before sunrise to run laps around the cement yard and do push-ups and sit-ups on the floor. I only found out later that 95 percent of female soldiers spend their active service sitting behind desks in offices, not firing guns. Still, we cocked our Uzis and learned how to load and unload a magazine and put together and dismantle a gun in three minutes and to make our beds, get dressed, and shower in five. At roll call at four in the morning, we stood at attention at the base of our beds, our berets resting on our shoulders, our boots laced up to the top, our shirts tucked in, our guns slung over our shoulders, and our mouths shut. Ready for inspection.

I hung out with Israeli girls who were military recruits training to defend their country in one of the most esteemed armies in the world. At night these same girls sat on their beds in their pajamas complaining that they were tired, hungry, or lazy, or they were missing their boyfriends, their mothers' cooking, and their beds. For me the physical side was not challenging, the exercise was not grueling, the superior officers' verbal abuse was not intimidating, the sleep deprivation was not painful, the fact that my Hebrew was limited to the vocabulary of a child was not disconcerting, and the food on which I binged was not disgusting. I acted the part in my combat uniform, smoking Marlboro cigarettes without filters and lying on my belly shooting real bullets at cardboard targets, not for one minute realizing the reality of my situation: that I was thousands of miles away from home training to become a soldier in the Israeli army. Nobody knew I was sick or realized that my bingeing was part of a serious disorder. If anybody had known that my very enrollment in the military was all just part of the illness, I would have been dismissed, discharged, and deported. Instead, I was treated like everybody else, even though I did not understand the orders and regulations because of the language barrier. I was even selected, along with four other girls, from two thousand, and driven out of the base camp on a number of occasions to perform seemingly asinine secret missions that we were forbidden to disclose to anybody. I only discovered at the end of basic training, after I was dismissed from the missions, that I had been on trial to join a division of the Army's Special Forces, but hadn't been accepted due to security reasons because I was a foreigner. Had I been accepted, I would have had to extend my army service and be sworn to a lifetime of total secrecy regarding my military undertakings.

At the end of the three weeks, however, as I was not destined to become an accidental secret agent, the officers in charge did not know where to place me in the system because my Hebrew was not good enough to do intelligence work. Instead of sending me to an *ulpan* to improve my Hebrew, for the first few months I sat every day on a bench at the central army base in town, aimlessly waiting for superior officers to decide what to do with someone like me who was not a volunteer but had not been reared all her life with a warfare mindset.

Before my recruitment, I had fantasized about the army. I had imagined barracks in a jungle with hammocks strewn between palm trees and soldiers in white sleeveless shirts, their dog tags shimmering in the sunlight. In truth, though, I hadn't given the reality much thought, and I wouldn't have been able to even if I had tried. I was subsequently relocated from base to base in an attempt to match me with something vaguely suitable. I was sent to the border of Lebanon, where I sat for twelve hours a day punching in the identity numbers of people entering and exiting Israel, then to a tiny base near the ocean where there were only six soldiers. Their mission had something to do with navigating for helicopters. But I couldn't understand a word nor grasp the concept, so I was relocated to a foreign liaison unit in Tel Aviv, although I did not know with whom the unit was liaising. I was out of my depth, out of my mind. Sick. Nobody knew I was deep in the crevices of a deadly disorder. They probably all thought I was just dumb, incapable, and a burden to the system.

Eventually my father intervened. He contacted a soldier he knew from his army service whose father was a high-ranking officer who could pull some strings. I remember visiting this officer and answering a couple of questions. Then he said, "What could you see yourself doing?" All I could think to say was, "I like to draw." He referred me to the education unit, located just outside of the city center, where they made documentaries. I stood every day behind a counter in what can only be described as a video store. I never watched a single film, didn't know what the documentaries were about, and had no idea what I was doing there, nor did I have the inclination to find out. Looking back, the situation was absurd. Life was a series of disconnected incidents that happened to me, over which I felt I had no power. I would remain there like a crazy patient in a psychiatric unit until dusk, when I would be dismissed to my father's home to sleep, only to return at dawn.

Months later, my father suddenly decided to leave the country for good and return to South Africa while I still had another nine months to spend in the army. Only years later did I find out that his business had liquidated and that he had been in a deep depression during that time. The day he left, which was soon after he disowned me, he handed me his checkbook and said it was just in case I needed money. I threw it back at his feet and told him I didn't need anything from him. In addition to my army day job, I was bartending at night, and I wanted to prove that I could survive on my own, that I could be independent and stable and capable. I wanted to prove that I could be in control of my life. I wanted to show him that his disowning me and abandoning me would not hurt me. I would prove that I felt nothing.

When he left, I packed up my belongings in the trunk of a second-hand car that my mother paid for after the Beetle died, and I slept at a rich friend's family house for a month, whose father worked for the Israeli mafia, living out of suitcases, and making out with her older brother in his basement bedroom. I was proving to myself that life was difficult. That nobody was there for me. That I wasn't worthy of stability and security. The fact that my mother called every other day from South Africa and begged me to come home meant nothing to me. That my father tried to get hold of me every week to make amends, but I ignored his calls, meant even less. I was determined to prove to the world that my life was hard. I didn't believe that I was worthy of more.

Usually when an Israeli soldier is alone in the country, what is officially known as a "lonely soldier," he or she receives financial compensation from the army as reimbursement for housing. But because I was a belated lonely soldier, since my father left the country more than halfway through my service, they refused to change my status, and I was not allowed to receive such compensation. The only money I had came from whatever I earned as a bartender at nights. After my army day job, I drove to the bar, changed out of my uniform in the car, and worked until two in the morning. Then I drove "home," slept four hours, and drove to the army base, where I fell asleep at my desk job. I charmed the customers at the bar at night and swore at my commanding officers in the army in the day. Instead of accepting money from the father I was resenting, I chose to do it on my own. How else could I justify the suffering, if I didn't call myself a victim?

In the army, I smashed chairs. I slammed doors. I cried. I had temper tantrums. But nobody ever asked me why. Maybe I wouldn't have had the answers. My superior officers just wrote me off like I was some kind of possessed cat. And I acted out like an angry and frustrated child by defying rules I thought were inane. I wore suede sneakers, which was forbidden, and left the top button of my shirt undone and my shirttails untucked, and walked around without my black beret folded over my shoulder and with my hair loose. It didn't help that my base was in a building located right next to the military police, all of whom patrolled the vicinity with clipboards, fining nonconformist soldiers like myself for violating army rules.

I got arrested for hitchhiking, interrogated by the military police, and punished with *rituk*, which involved detention on weekends, where I guarded a gate in the dead of night. I woke up throughout the night, every few hours, to stand in front of a gate and let visitors in and out. Then I crawled back into the metal bunk bed with my gun because I was told that if I let it out of my sight, I would be incarcerated for seven years, no questions asked. Once I had accumulated nine fines to my name for all my disobediences, I stood trial in an official military court for violation of the rules. The last fine was for wearing my suede sneakers. I was acquitted because I couldn't understand the sentencing and there was no one to translate it into English. Even though I had learned to read and write Hebrew better than I had when I was recruited, the language was still a struggle. But I was more used to it that way. No matter how hard it was, I chose to endure. I refused to give up.

At the beginning of my last year of service, the unit's secretary, a well-groomed, ladylike, simpleminded, and complaisant Russian girl, completed her service. I took over her position and tried to emulate her in an attempt to attain her easygoing nature. I tried to sit calmly behind my desk answering phones and manicuring my nails. I lined up bottles of nail polish and cuticle remover and emery boards, and I filed and glossed and buffed every day. And every half hour, I went to the restroom to take a pee and get a coffee from the vending machine and a cigarette from my pack. I sat in the corridor alternating one sip of my coffee with one puff of my cigarette. Sip. Puff. Sip. Puff. Sip. Puff. Sip. And when the cup was empty and my bladder full and I had smoked the cigarette down to the butt, I waited for another half hour to pass before taking another pee, getting another coffee, and smoking another cigarette. This daily ritual made me feel like my life had order and purpose, no matter how small and insignificant, as long as I got it right every single time.

I was still staying in the family home of a friend, the Israeli mafia member's daughter, whose best friend was an anorexic visiting from London. To me, she was a real anorexic. She was stick thin, bony and tanned, and her face was so gaunt that her teeth jutted out and her eyes bulged. Her straw hair was long and straight and died blonde with peroxide. She was on vacation, and she seemed carefree and oblivious to the fact that she was dying. I wanted to be just like her. But I wasn't. I woke up every morning at six to get to the army on time while she got up at noon to go to the beach. I had real responsibilities while all she was doing was tanning. I worked every night after my army shift to pay my way while she had a bottomless budget that she spent on alcohol, cigarettes, and tropical tanning oil. I envied her so much. Nothing seemed to faze her. I didn't realize at the time that this was only because she was so deep in the disorder of anorexia nervosa that she was half dead. But I just wanted some of that "ease."

For the two weeks that she was in town, I shadowed her. When I had any time off, we lay tanning on deck chairs on the beach, wearing sneakers with our bikinis. We drank Diet Cokes and smoked Camel Lights. The combination tasted vile. But the idea of it felt cool. "You know you are too thin," I said. "You know that if you don't put on some weight, you'll be infertile, right?" She stared ahead and puffed on her cigarette. And the more I nagged, the more she smoked. "Denial will kill you," I said, lighting up another cigarette and sipping my Diet Coke. Later, in her room, I sat on the edge of her guest bed and watched her skinny body angled at her dressing table, one bony knee hoisted up on the chair as she smeared cocoa-butter lotion fastidiously all over her bronzed matchstick legs. I watched her as though she would lather me with some of her "wisdom" so I would know how to make my own pain go away.

As soon as she returned to London, I carried on emulating her in every superficial way: wearing sneakers to the beach, smoking the same brand of cigarettes as she did, and drinking only Diet Coke. I even bought the same cocoa-butter lotion and applied it to my body several times a day in the hope that my pale skin would shine. A few months later, on the day I turned twenty, I would stop eating, again. This time it would be a conscious decision. I hated putting on weight from all the bingeing in the army cafeteria, where I ate double or triple portions of everything. I hated that other girls were thinner than me, and I hated myself more and more each day for hating myself. I wanted, more than anything, what that British anorexic girl had.

I still believed that being Ana would someday make me happy. (In the eating disorder world, Ana is a nickname for anorexia.)

When my mom found out that I was living out of a suitcase and crashing at different people's houses, and that I absolutely refused to come home, she arranged for me to move in with Tia, an old friend of hers, a dance instructor, who had three sons in their early twenties. Although Tia took me in like one of her own, she still had a full house, so she cleared a corner in the open-plan kitchen-cum-living room and put down a single mattress for my bed. She cleared the kitchen broom cupboard so that I had somewhere to put my clothes, and I stashed my underwear in a shoebox at the head of the mattress. The boys jostled in with their friends in the early hours of the morning with cologne bodies, beer breath, and Marlboro voices, and I lay there on my mattress on the kitchen floor, in my silky G-string, entangled in the sheets, wanting them to lust after me. Wanting them to love me. I didn't know the difference.

At the time, my self-destructive mindset had been going on for six years without any successful intervention or respite. But this was just the beginning. On my twentieth birthday, I ate only a packet of crackers and a yogurt. Then every day after that, for two weeks, I ate only ice cream. I was once again on a downward spiral of weight loss. Over the months, I went through phases of eliminating different foods. I had become an expert at telling myself that I loved everything I hated and hated everything I loved. I said that I didn't need to lose weight but that I loved being stick thin. I loved the feeling. But it would take me years to understand that thin is not a feeling.

Tia told me years later that she had tried to talk to me many times about my restrictive, destructive eating behavior but I don't remember any of it. An anorexic mind has an amazing way of blocking out help. What I do remember, because I still have them, is that I began to purge my thoughts in secret journals that I would end up keeping rather than burning.

I'd better eat, or I'll collapse. I cannot become obsessive again. It's too time-wasting. I'm so irritable. I don't know what the fuck is wrong with me. Time just goes by, and I don't feel it. I feel nothing. I feel like doing nothing. I feel like nothing. What the fuck is wrong with me? It's just not worth it sometimes—the struggle of survival. I have no reason to feel like this. But I can't stop it. It's just here. It arrives and remains dormant. I feel like I'm going insane. I cannot be on my own. I cannot be like this on my own. What is happening to me? Why do I feel this way? This is all life is—waiting for time to go by.

I feel like lying under this duvet forever. I feel like smoking the joint in my cupboard. Something weird is happening to me. My head is spinning. I feel like doing drugs. I read an article on anorexia nervosa. The definition it gave is a constant striving to lose weight. I am like this. I don't eat normally, but I'm not underweight. What the fuck is normal? I'm not depressed. I'm not happy. I'm not even in between. I'm nowhere. It said anorexia nervosa is a biological predisposition toward a societal something or other. In other words, it is a need to be in control. It's not a desire to be thin. It is a personality change, an emotional change, not a bodily change. It is not an aesthetic disease. It's a disease of the mind. Those who die played the sick game to the end and lost. Because inevitably you lose. Nobody can beat it. Nobody.

I can't survive on coffee and cigarettes. I need to change this to a healthier lifestyle, otherwise I'll die. Everyone is gnawing at my head that I'm skinny enough and that if I continue I'll die. I don't want to be this way. A food fanatic. A calorie counter. A weight-obsessive person. I don't need to go through this hell again. I'm not stupid. I can beat it sensibly this time. I need only to alter my thoughts. To per-

suade myself that I need to eat healthy. To eliminate the aftertaste and the guilt. To keep watching my weight so I don't get paranoid. I need sustenance because otherwise it's a simple fact: I'll die. And I don't want to at all.

This is what I want to be like: She eats very little / She never takes second helpings / She never stuffs her face / She never finishes what's on her plate / She never eats fattening food / She occasionally eats a junk meal / She doesn't smoke excessively / She never snacks between meals / She's always gracious / She's always clean and fresh / She's bony and healthy-looking / She always knows what to order / If she doesn't like it, she doesn't eat it.

The saddest part of what I wrote that day was that I honestly had no idea what was going on with me. It wasn't ignorance or stupidity. It was anorexia. Denial. Distortion. Disorder. I convinced myself that everything was fine, and the fact that I still clung to my father's disowning me and I was sleeping on a mattress in a kitchen, surviving on ice cream, was no indication to me that I was in dire straits. I should have listened to myself when I said I felt insane. I was. My behavior warranted institutionalization. Instead, it was overlooked or punished. No officer or soldier took me aside to tell me that I was out of control and needed help. Nobody thought pain was at the root of my anger. But I was so entrenched in the sickness, I would not have listened anyway, especially not to authority. I was on my own mission. I was high on adrenaline and concentrating on not putting anything in my body. It was hard work; it was survival, and it kept me going. It kept me oblivious. I was so out of touch with my body and with how I was feeling. And I couldn't stop. That was the scariest thing for me. Anorexia was like being on a life-support machine—it kept me going, that control. In my mind, it was the only thing protecting me.

A few months before my release from the army, I was promoted in rank from corporal to sergeant, while at home I was promoted from the kitchen floor to one of the boy's rooms after he moved out. The domestic move only gave me more privacy, on which anorexia thrived, and on the military front, the third stripe on my insignia only meant I was getting closer to the end. And with no hopes, plans, or dreams ahead, this scared me. I turned, in extreme, to the only thing I had come to rely on to make me feel safe over the years. I cut out all foods except grapes and popcorn. My body had figured out that I needed the sugar and carbohydrates. Every day on my way to the army, I drove to the same grocery store and bought a pound of green grapes and ate them one by one over the course of the day, in between my coffee sipping and cigarette smoking. Twelve hours later, I drove home, and, as long as nobody was around, I prepared my dinner.

I stashed a small bag of popcorn kernels in the kitchen cupboard that I replenished regularly, and night after night, I used a teaspoon of oil to cook a full pot of popcorn for myself. Afterward, I cleaned the counter and the stove and opened the windows so there would be no trace of it. I tucked the kernels in the back of the cupboard behind all the cans so that nobody noticed it. And then I dumped the popped popcorn into a round plastic bowl for kneading dough and doused it with salt. I snuck off to my room, shut the door behind me, closed the shutters so it was dark as fear, and sat cross-legged on the bed, wrapping my legs around the huge bowl in my lap.

While other people my age were out gallivanting around the city, celebrating their youth, meeting at coffee shops, dancing in clubs, listening to live music, and eating out, I was home alone sneaking popcorn. I watched MTV on a low volume so that I would hear the front door open. I sat there for hours in the dark, night after night, on my own, eating my popcorn one kernel at a time and watching mind-deadening music videos. It was an addiction. A ritual. As long as I was there, I felt safe. Contained. It was sadder and more pathetic than doing hard drugs. Doing popcorn. Everyone eats popcorn at the movies. Together. As a snack. Between meals. I ate it alone. As my dinner. Night after night. For three months. It was my fix.

Every night, Tia and I played this game where she would come home and knock on my door and ask, "Have you eaten yet?" Every time, I said, "Yes." Then she would go away and leave me alone with myself. But one night when she knocked on my door and asked if I'd eaten yet and I said yes, instead of going away, she pushed open my door and saw me sitting there with the plastic bowl on my lap. She walked into my secret.

"I'm sorry to barge in like this," she said, "but I asked my son if you had eaten, and he said sarcastically, 'Yes, a whole bite of lettuce!' So I have come here to tell you that I am sick and tired of your behavior! If you want to kill yourself, just do it quickly because I do not have the patience for this. I have tried to talk to you so many times about your diet and self-destruction, but you don't hear me. I can't watch you slowly dying in my house anymore. Do you hear me?"

She sat down slowly on the edge of my bed, and I moved back a little so my back was against the wall.

"I'm sorry," I said, lowering my head to look down into the bowl. The dry popcorn kernels looked like extracted decayed teeth with gold fillings.

"Do you have any idea what this is doing to your body? Do you think I don't know that you eat nothing? I haven't wanted to tell your mother because she would worry sick, she would be on the first plane here. I don't know what to tell her."

Tia looked around my cave as though it were the first time she had seen darkness.

"I know, I'm sorry," I said in a whisper. "I know this is not good for me, but I don't care about myself anymore. I just don't."

"Well let me tell you, my girl, that this 'diet' you are on is nothing but self-destruction! Many of my dancers suffer from eating disorders. One dancer's sister died from anorexia."

She moved back a little and asked if she could open the blinds. I nodded yes.

"She died?" I asked Tia while she still had her back to me.

"Yes! This is no joke. You are playing with your life! Do you understand that?"

It was dusk outside, and I heard crickets chirping and felt a breeze blowing through the blinds. Tia sat down again and aimed the remote control at the TV and switched it off. A soft glow filled the room.

"I know it's really hurting my family, especially my mom . . ."

"She is worried sick about you, child! She calls me all the time begging me to ask you to go home and get well," she said, patting my knee bone.

"I know it's not healthy, but I've gone too far to . . ."

"Listen, I'm surprised at how aware you are of your behavior, but I can also see that you still don't understand how far you have actually taken this and how serious it is. I hate to say this, but if you don't get your act together soon, young lady, you will die."

"I'll try," I whispered, tucking my chin into my chest.

Tia stood up. "Thank you for opening up to me tonight. After all this time, I didn't think you would be willing to talk. And I'm sorry if I came down on you too hard; I appreciate that you weren't angry with me."

I glanced down at the popcorn kernels and felt that same old blockage in my throat and knot in my stomach. The room was quiet, and I heard children's laughter outside. She walked to the door and turned to say, "You can feel free to talk to me any time. You know that, right? Please, whatever you do, don't bottle it up. We all love you so much. You are like a daughter to me."

She closed the door. I sat clasping my bowl, staring into the abyss of loneliness.

Someday, I will have to have a meal at a table surrounded by people.

Chapter Eleven

RAVE BUNNY

In the army, the soldiers talked more about drugs than they did about war or peace. They talked about hallucinations on acid, the best sex of their lives on ecstasy (more commonly called *E*), and the interconnected universe on magic mushrooms. While they shared their stories, I marked off the days until my release with Xs on the wall next to my desk. When there were one hundred Xs, I was discharged from the Israel Defense Force. A sergeant. Free. I handed in my gun, gave back my shirt with its three-striped insignia, and fled, just like I had done as a child, only this time it was voluntary and I would not look back.

By that time, I felt that I had overstayed my welcome in Tia's home. And I had awoken from my lifelong dream of becoming an Israeli. By the end of my service, the army, for me, was no longer about belonging, like it had been when I was conscripted. It was only about endurance. I felt compelled to prove to myself that if I could endure, if I could push through no matter how challenging, boring, or frustrating, then it would mean that I had survived, even if all I was surviving on were grapes and popcorn.

Three days after my discharge, I was on a plane back to

South Africa. I had run the race and reached the finish line. A winner. My army friends moved on to real jobs, while the only thing that lay in my path was the hope of scoring recreational drugs so I could belong to a carefree subculture about which I had heard so much. I would no longer have to be responsible for guns, answer to people with power on their shoulders, or wake up at the crack of dawn to guard a gate. I had a new purpose. I was determined to become a VIP of the drug underworld. I fell into it as if it were the deepest and darkest of mines.

Once I was back in dangerous, depressing Johannesburg, my mother and I found ourselves living together in her old house, just the two of us. All the lodgers had left, and my sister had moved to Cape Town soon after she had completed high school. I moved into my sister's old room, which was next door to my mother's. She wanted to lie next to me and hold my hand while I poured out my feelings about my experiences, my transition, and what really happened in the last few years of this critical time in my young life in a foreign land with a father who had said he disowned me, but was calling me every other day now that I was back in South Africa, again to make amends but still, I was refusing his calls. She wanted to know everything.

But I said nothing. Despite the pain my mother felt for not being able to save her own daughter, she still had the sweetest smile and eyes like a child who knows no evil. I had dead hair, zero vitality, and eyes that showed no feeling. For the two months that my mom and I lived together, I was only "nice" to her when I wanted to borrow her car to go to the gym and burn my "fat" at aerobics classes or to go to the rave clubs to burn my brain on drugs, dancing, and pounding music. As soon as I was confronted with the words *eating disorder, thin, angry, self-centered,* or *hungry,* I slammed my door shut and retreated into my narrow, illusory world of abstention and deprivation, my world without food.

On my first night back I got ready for bed in my sister's room. She had left behind a closetful of old clothes she didn't need anymore. I found her silk pajama pants with pink roses that she had worn every night before I left. The elastic was stretched out, and the seams came apart. I ran my hand over the soft material and cradled it in my arms. I reached into the cupboard for a T-shirt, and my mother opened the door.

"Mom! I told you to knock!" I yelled, covering my chest with both arms.

I stood still in my baggy panties, hugging my body tight. My mother stared at me and cupped her mouth with her hands. She let out a gasp and shook her head from side to side while pacing up and down like a madwoman saying, "No no no no no no . . ." At last she pulled herself together enough to say, "You are so thin," she said. "Tia told me not to be shocked when I saw you, but I didn't realize. You are much too thin! Much much much too thin . . ."

"I told you to knock!" I shouted. She ignored me and kept staring and shaking her head like I was a cut in one of her canvases.

"Mom, I am talking to you! I don't want you to barge in like this anymore!"

She stared at my stomach, and her button eyes looked like they were going to pop.

"What is that thing in your stomach?" I looked down. I had forgotten it was there. "What have you done to yourself? There is a piece of metal in your belly button!"

"It's called a piercing, Mom! A belly ring. And for your information, there is nothing wrong with it. Everyone has one."

"I can't believe you did that to yourself! When? Why?"

"Oh, Jesus, leave me alone, it's no big deal." I slipped into the pajama pants and turned my back on her to pull on my T-shirt.

"Are you smoking?" she asked.

"No! I have not been smoking!" I lied. "And so what if I was? It's none of your business!"

She paced back and forth with one hand on her hip and the other covering her eyes.

"You are destroying yourself," she said. "You are wasting away. All your beauty, your innocence . . . You are as thin as a rake. It's pathetic! I can't see you going downhill like this again, because that is where you are headed: downhill. Do you hear me? Downhill."

"If I disturb you so much, then don't look! Leave. Me. Alone! I don't need a lecture! I've done nothing wrong! And don't call me pathetic!"

"Where is the exquisite, delicate being you once were? Where is she?"

Her tears sat on her eyelashes like dewdrops about to plop off blades of grass.

I stood stiff as a wire. "Get out! There is nothing wrong with me! Just leave me alone!"

I shooed her away with my hand as though she were a messenger with unwanted news. She backed away and closed the door. But a second later she opened it and stormed back in.

"You have no right! How long is this going to go on for? I told you that the army and being away from your home and living with your fucking father would damage you! I begged you to come home, but you were adamant. Adamant! Like you always are . . ."

"Get out!" I yelled, stamping my feet on the ground.

"I don't know what to do for you anymore! I just want my daughter back! Is that too much to ask?"

She slammed the door behind her. I sucked in my breath and covered my ears. *Fuck fuck fuck.* I grabbed a sweatshirt out of the cupboard and wrapped it around my body leaving the zipper undone. I leaned out the open window, lit a cigarette, pulled the sweatshirt tighter around me, and stared out the window, puffing away like it was my last cigarette on my dying day.

This eating thing. My weight varies during the day. I know I'm thin, yet I don't see myself as skinny. I cannot consume food no matter what it is without feeling guilt and hatred toward myself—for losing control, for enjoying. After consumption I feel the need to starve myself or deprive myself of what foods comprise my "forbidden" list. Today I had a salad with feta cheese and five squares of chocolate. I can't get this off my mind. The guilt. I can feel it building inside me. I can't do this. It's all gone wrong. Surely there are more important things to concentrate on. Maybe I just won't eat anything and then I will never feel guilty. I won't eat unless it's offered to me. I won't crave anything. I won't prepare my own meals. I won't eat. Only when there's food placed in front of me, cooked for everyone, and I have to join, because I can't always run away, will I eat. Then I'll eat only the non-fattening things, and I won't finish what's on my plate, and I won't go for seconds, and I won't eat between meals, and I won't drink coffee one cup after the other, and I won't have five teaspoons of sugar in every cup. I will drink more water. No chocolate. Is this normal? I just can't get it right!

I want a diet that will allow me to eat the very minimum of everything but still receive the proper nutrients for my body, growth, health, repair, functioning. I don't want my hair to fall out or my periods to stop again or to be anemic or anything like that. And I don't want to put on any weight. If I fluctuate, it must only be down. I don't care if I eat very little as long as I'm getting enough of the proper nutrients. I want to cut out some things and force others. I want to be given rules —allowed or forbidden—otherwise I lose control. I need these restrictions, these laws, these tests, these challenges. Otherwise I can do anything.

This gives me boundaries to live by; I decide to make or break them, and I suffer the consequences. It's my body, and nobody can stop me or force me. It's my own choice. What I put in MY mouth is MY business and no one else's. The bigger you are, the more you are prone to challenges. Small makes you vulnerable, unchallenged, but protected by this look. It's your shield because underneath you are not indestructible, yet with this look you cannot be defeated or violated because you are uninviting aesthetically and so no one would want to hurt you.

One of the ironies about anorexia is that you work so hard to harden yourself in an attempt to protect yourself from pain yet you don't register that by conforming to anorexia's "norms" you are hurting yourself every step of the way by the very nature of the disorder. That's why you easily fall for anything that disguises itself as happiness. Even if it's a false happiness so small that you can hold it in the palm of your hand.

Exactly one week after I was discharged from the army and living back in South Africa, I hooked up with a girl I knew who was plugged into the rave scene. Her name was Porsche, and she invited me to go with her to a rave at a massive warehouse called the Furnace in an obscure place on the outskirts of Johannesburg. Her mother made us special outfits for the occasion. Hers was bright blue Lycra leggings with one leg cut off at the knee like shorts and a purple crop top with pixie sleeves. Mine was a luminous orange Lycra catsuit.

Porsche and I waited in line at the rave. She told me to cup my hand and plopped two white ecstasy pills in my palm.

"Swallow," she said. "Tonight you gonna be double dropping!"

One pill had a Superman stamp on it and the other an engraving of a peace dove. I swigged them down with a caffeinated energy juice and waited for them to kick in. An hour later, we rubbed against wet bodies pulsating to flashing strobes and darting laser beams. Hundreds of rave bunnies thumped to the hard beat of house music, and Porsche asked me if I was "rushing."

"What?"

"Are you feeling it?"

My lower back is hot / it pinches / the back of my neck tingles / my forehead and my cheeks are numb / my eyes are open wide / color everywhere / I see music / the beat is manic / raging / my legs are heavy but my moves are light as air / I feel happy and alive and happy to be alive / my mind is empty / I think of nothing / my lips are swelling / I'm grinding my teeth and biting my lips and chewing like a mad cow / I can't stop dancing / jumping / pounding / screaming / I can't stop moving / I can't stop smiling / E N E R G Y / arms up in the air / I'm screaming / AAAAAAAAAHHHHHHH / YES! Oh my GOD this is amazingggggggggggggggggg / my back is hot / my neck is tingling / my eyes are rolling back / I can feel the music inside me all around me up and over through me surging purging / my face is crawling / I'm screaming / YES! / I must be dreaming / I have never in all my life felt so fuckingggggggg happyyyyyyyyyyy!

A rave bunny was the perfect persona for an anorexic. Perfect armor. I could be skinny and skittish and frenetic and absent-minded and blame it on being a rave bunny. And rave bunnies don't eat. They suck lollipops. They gulp down loads of energy drinks. They wear skimpy tight bright fluorescent synthetic clothes that hug their bones. They go mad. They lose it. They let go because they're high on ecstasy. There is only one rule for rave bunnies: keep dancing. And it became my scapegoat. I lost weight. Blamed it on the dancing. I danced twelve hours straight. Blamed it on E. The drug made starving easy because it erased my appetite. The high made me feel invincible. Raving was an exaggerated extension of my aerobics high. Raving gave me the same release as aerobics, and dropping E made it a thousand times greater.

One night I sat next to a guy in the chill-out zone at the rave club who boasted to his bunny buddies that, over the months, he had taken one hundred Es. *What an achievement*, I thought. *I want to be just like him.* To say I've reached the one-hundred mark. It was another cross-addiction for sure—one that was especially alluring because it swallowed my mind, drowned my thoughts, and made me feel like the happiest person alive in this fluffy, infantile, pacifier-sucking, lollipop-licking, bouncy smiley happy baby world. But when the music died down and the comedown kicked in, it all came rushing back. Worse. Everyone went home to their mundane routines to face the piercing daylight and the nauseating sun. When you are a nocturnal animal, it is easy to forget reality.

And then all I can think of, while pounding my feet on the empty dance floor, is my own insignificance. I take a step away from myself and see someone with a good heart, an intelligent mind, a deep soul, someone creative and artistic and talented, with a beautiful physique who is wrecking herself from the outside in. And I rub her out. In her place is a lost freak forever going through pathetic identity crises, unworthy of anything good or positive. Undeserving. Because she is a failure. She is repulsive because she is a fake. And they lock in a tug-of-war. The feelings in her heart and the intuition of her soul have not yet been cultivated. She is waiting to be adopted by kindness, love, and tenderness. Because she shoves all her hatred deep inside and everyone can smell this rotting mess. She has taught herself to deny beauty, to ignore sensitivity, to be hard and manipulative in order to survive, but she is shallow and boring, and she will end up a reject because she does not realize her own worth.

My mom made many attempts during those months to reach out to me. She had seen a documentary on TV about girls suffering with anorexia nervosa, and she was determined that I watch it. She called the broadcaster and begged them to screen it again, but they wouldn't. Eventually she managed to track down someone at the station who said they would make a VHS copy of the program for her to collect. She coerced me into driving with her to the gate of someone's house in some suburb, and they passed it through the bars to her.

Days later, I was watching TV on the couch, and she walked in and slotted the video into the machine and asked me, please, to stay. Before I could say no, I was watching what, according to the narrator, was an informative look into the private lives of a small group of severely malnourished anorexic girls at a private clinic in Canada run by one woman with an undying passion to save these girls. I watched it with a vacant expression on my face, bored, as though I were watching the weather report, or golf. My mother wanted me to be shocked. To recoil in horror. To empathize to the point of tears. But to me it was just a bunch of forlorn characters moping. *These girls are dying, they are on their deathbeds, they have wasted away to nothing!* was what my mom wanted me to say. Instead, I said they were nothing like me.

That was all that my mom found back then, in 1996, to appeal to me, to encourage me to relate to my self-destruction. Nowadays, there are hundreds of books out there; there are videos on the Internet. It's in the media; it makes the news. Activists are advocating against it, and there are organizations opposed to it, educating and empowering the public with knowledge of anorexia's destructive results. But in those days, in South Africa, there was nothing but some documentary on public TV, never to be screened again.

She tried to get me to watch the Oprah episode where Oprah interviewed some girls about their bodies and image and vanity. I sat eating lettuce and tomatoes with no dressing and gazing up at the show, disinterested and detached. I thought that by acquiescing to her demands, I was placidly getting her off my back. Still, my mom was on a mission to prove to me the consequences of my ways. She talked me into going to a psychologist. I went once or twice and told my mother it did nothing for me. She also took me to a woman who may have been a dietician. I remember she weighed me and I lay almost stark naked on her table but I don't recall anything else about that meeting. I had no idea what I was doing there and as far as I could tell, nothing came of that either. Doctors of all kinds were blind to the signs and symptoms I was involuntarily presenting. They sent me home after inadequate appraisals, their ignorance speaking louder than their words. They had no clue that my noncompliance and indifference were blatant clues to my disorder.

My mom then took me to a kinesiologist, who decided I was fine but gave me a protein-shake supplement to drink instead of eating meals. It came in a huge white container like diet whey powder. I could choose from three flavors. I chose vanilla. I drank that shake every morning and afternoon and sometimes in the evening at the kitchen table out of the same pear-shaped milkshake glass. I loved the ritual of measuring the powder, adding the water, and carefully stirring in exactly five spoonfuls of artificial sweetener. It made me feel like I was receiving special treatment. It was like prescription medicine, and it made me feel safe. It was my placebo food. I had always wished that I had to take medicine or that I had an allergy that forbade me to eat certain foods. I think I really just needed some boundaries.

One night, I was sitting in the kitchen in my sister's rose pajamas drinking my dinnertime protein shake in my milkshake glass, and my mom stormed in ranting and raving. She stood in the doorway waving a finger at me and screamed, "You are a selfish bitch!"

I put my glass down and wrapped both hands around it. I hunched my shoulders and retreated into my shell.

"Do you know what you are aspiring to? Do you? No, you have no fucking idea that you are well on your way to becoming like all the shits out there!" she said.

It was the first time in my life that I was scared of my mother. "Get dressed," she said. "I'm taking you to a bar."

"I don't want to go to some bar. I don't feel like it."

"Why?" She put on her most sarcastic tone and pretended to be applying make-up and doing up her hair. "Isn't there enough time to make yourself, your hair, your body beautiful?"

I looked down, and every muscle in my body tensed up. I thought she was going to hit me, but instead she mocked me.

"Why? Isn't it as good as a rave club?" she screamed at the top of her voice, and her eyes had madness in them and she stumbled over her feet. I kept completely still and looked down.

She carries on mocking me and criticizing what I do. For what? I have nothing to say. I'm holding my milkshake glass, staking out my position.

She acted out the scenario between us: "Kiss . . . love you . . . borrowing your car . . . going out . . . rave rave rave . . . kiss . . . love you . . . rave rave rave . . . It's so bloody fake that it makes me sick!" she spat. She waved her arms and acted out the scene again like a pantomime. "Either I am going to bury an emaciated child, or you are going to bury an exhausted mother!" she yelled at the top of her voice, poking her finger into her chest and waving it back at me.

I had never seen my mother irate. I sat tight, trying to think of an escape route.

What if she kills me? I should call my sister. I need help. She's

going to hurt me. I need to escape. Mommy's gone stark raving mad.
I'm scared she's going to hurt me.

She stormed out screaming and slamming doors. A few minutes later she stumbled back in.

"I hate you!" she yelled, clutching a whiskey bottle. "You are slowly killing yourself! Don't you see that if you carry on this way, you are going to die? I love you! Why are you doing this? You are going to kill yourself! I can't take it . . . I can't take it . . ."

I can't deal with this. I don't lay my shit on her. So what if I find it hard to communicate sometimes? So what if I find it difficult to show affection? Kill me for it. I'm not so fucking evil. I'm just minding my own business. What the fuck is wrong with her? Why must she be so mad at me? I never tried to hurt her. I only want her to be happy. I'm sorry if I can't give her happiness. I'm so sorry to disappoint her. You would think I'm a fucking junkie, crackhead, bitch, whore, loser the way she carries on. There are worse kids in this world. Maybe if there were some rules in this fucking house I'd have been more obedient. This time I won't scream. I won't answer back. I don't think I'm disrespectful. I'm not trying to spite. I can't handle this shit. I can't see my mother like this. I'll just back off. I'll back off. And it's all inside me. And I won't let it out. She's fucking schizophrenic. She screams she hates me then says she loves me then she hates me then she loves me.

"I don't want you anywhere near me! I don't want to fucking see your face! Just get away from me! I don't want you near me!" she screamed. "I'm leaving! I'm going drinking! I'm going out to get a life so that I don't have to look after you all the fucking time!"

What the fuck have I done? I just want to run away run away run away run away.

She stormed out. I heard the ignition start, and she reversed out the driveway, screeching the tires like a maniac.

I hope she doesn't kill herself. I can't stop her because she's a grown woman and she can do whatever she wants.

I got up to call my sister, but I couldn't get hold of her. Ten minutes later, my mother was back. The front door slammed. She swung open the cupboard door and grabbed another whiskey bottle off the top shelf.

"I don't want you near me! I'm going upstairs to bed because you drive me to fucking drink! Literally!"

What the fuck is she taking the whiskey bottle with her to bed for? She's going to kill herself soon.

"I will commit suicide if you carry on like this! I mean it! I will kill myself!"

Is it really because of me? Am I so bad? What have I done? What haven't I done? I don't need this shit. I can't handle it. Rave rave rave rave rave rave rave rave rave.

"Your life is not so bad!" she said over and over again.

I never said it was. I'm actually having a good time sometimes. I love raving. I love E. I'm not suffering day in and day out. She is. She's suffering for my pain because she chooses to. I don't need to go stark raving mad like she does to express my fucking emotions. I'm different from my mother. It's my choice if I want to block it out, become distant, and put up defenses. This is my way of dealing with it. I am me.

My mother slammed the cupboard door shut, and I heard her glug down the whiskey. She must have stood for a few seconds at the bottom of the stairway thinking about whether to make another entrance. Instead, she stormed upstairs, and I prayed that in the morning, when I woke, she would not be drunk and passed out. Or worse.

I don't even think it's about weight. I looked great before. I said I'd lose a few pounds and then never stopped wanting to lose. Now I'm on the border. If I lose nine more pounds, then I've hit rock bot-

tom. I hope I do. Then I'd keep it that way. And yes, it's all about numbers for me because numbers don't lie. Who are you to judge what I look like, what weight I should be, how I look best or worst? It's my decision. It's my body, and you may have to look at it or close your eyes and turn away, but I have to live in it. I don't know if it's about this because I dig food. I dig the taste, but I hate to think about it. I've managed to confuse my own body. It doesn't know when to be hungry or thirsty anymore. It can't trust itself. My mind is torn by health, fertility, normality, and achieving my unattainable goal of self-obliteration—purity, nothingness, the ultimate. I'm now standing on the edge trying to balance, and my mind is unsteady. It doesn't want to turn either way for fear of getting worse, but it can't hold on much longer. Why is holding on easier than letting go?

If I let go, then what? I can get fat, enjoy, be myself, fear, rejection, guilt. If I hold on I can grip and try to pull myself up so that I'm sitting on top, out of reach, out of sight, on a high, narrow wall waiting till it's safe or till someone comes to rescue me. The way up is much less than the way down—down is a steep fall, and up is a hard step, but it's secure if you reach it. Down you never know what may happen on the way, how long it'll take, and where you'll land when you reach the ground. I can't figure this out at all. Maybe I'm just so vain and empty all I want is to be thin, grossly thin. What the fuck is this about? Why won't I allow myself to eat? Food, health, fuel. Why, why, why? I don't want to end up in a hospital or lose my periods again. I don't want to eat all I can. I don't want to gain weight. I don't want sometimes to be in this body that has let me down, humiliated me, made me ashamed.

I didn't know then that after midnight, on the night of our fight, my mother had called a rehabilitation clinic. A nurse answered. My mother said, "I am lost . . . I'm beside myself . . . I don't know what to do anymore . . . is there any help I can get? Must I bring her in? Please help me . . . My daughter has not

eaten in years . . . she is not well . . ." I didn't know this. All I
saw was that a couple of days later, she seemed to have calmed
down. She still allowed me to borrow her car. She also still
looked at me with that "I've done her wrong" look. And I still
went out every night to party, to rave, to let rip, to get high, to
get happy. I still came home at sunrise and slept and went to the
gym and out to party again.

Before leaving the house on my way to the club one night, I
went upstairs to say goodbye and to reassure her that what I was
doing was right.

"I'm borrowing your car, Mom, okay? Don't worry about
me, and don't wait up for me. I'll be home later, I don't know
what time. Okay?"

She lay dead still on her back under the covers with the duvet
pulled up to her neck. I leaned over to kiss her quick on the cheek.

"I called Tara," she said softly in a stifled voice. I retreated
from her bed. I knew that Tara was a rehabilitation clinic for
girls with bulimia and anorexia, and I had heard stories in school
that it was like a prison and that the girls counted the days until
they got out. In Tara, girls were weighed, force-fed, and treated
like caged animals.

"For what? Tara is a lunatic asylum!" I shouted. In that moment, it felt as if my own mother had stabbed me in the back
with the Bedouin knife she kept hidden under her bed. "Raving
is what is making me lose weight," I said in an icy voice. "That's
all!" She looked ahead, ignoring me, like I had no right to talk.
"You try dancing all night and see what happens to your body!
All teenagers go clubbing, Mom! There is nothing wrong with
me! Don't you get that?"

"I am warning you," she said in a tone that I had never before heard from her, a tone of discipline and authority. "If you
do not start eating properly, I will send you to Tara."

I stepped back and looked at her. *This woman is supposed to be my mother. This woman is supposed to love me. This woman is not supposed to betray me.* Not until years later would I understand that my mother was trying with all her might to save me. Not until years later would I understand that the impetus behind her "betrayal" was undying love and not absolute cruelty.

What have I done to myself? The doctors say that if I continue to eat and exercise like this and rave on E that I can drop dead from cardiac arrest. A heart attack! My head is in turmoil. They all think I'm pathetic and weak and are completely worried. I can't take it anymore. I don't want to die like this. I love E. Our family is going to fall apart. I need to stop this shit. I don't know what to do. I feel like escaping for a long time. I am losing my mind. I feel insane. I can't live like this anymore. Fuck! I'm not being honest with myself. Am I really anorexic? I don't want this disease. I want to fight it. Beat it. Get rid of it . . . But I love E.

Around the same time that my mother had called Tara, she had also been referred to a man called Rob, the father of two daughters who had survived eating disorders, who then dedicated his life to helping other sufferers. One day she called him behind my back to beg his advice. He said to her: "Your daughter is sick. She has a serious illness. It is called anorexia."

She tells me it was the first time that someone else had acknowledged how bad my disorder was and that she knew I needed to be made aware of this or she might lose me. My mother knew that I would refuse her help or any kind of family intervention, so she tried casually to get me to respond to his call so that it would not seem as though she had conspired against me by wanting with all her heart and soul to save my life.

The phone call came about a week after she told me she

would send me to Tara. I was sitting at the foot of my sister's bed wearing her silky rose pajamas, drinking my vanilla protein shake with five sweeteners in my milkshake glass for lunch. My mother knocked tentatively.

"There is someone on the phone who would like to speak to you about where you are at," she said softly.

She purposefully avoided using words like *anorexia, disorder,* or *eating problem* because it evoked rage in me. Up until that point, I had barely uttered any of those words aloud, especially to my mother.

"Is that okay?" she asked.

"Fine!" I shouted.

She tiptoed in, tugging at the long telephone cord that dragged behind her. She handed me the phone and left the room.

I spoke with Rob that day for two hours, but I don't remember a single word we said. I don't even remember the gist of the conversation. What I do remember is that he wasn't soft with me. He wasn't sympathetic. He expressed no pity. No sadness. He was authoritative. Firm. He put the cards on the table. He had to, otherwise I would not have opened up to him. Anorexia doesn't respond to kindness. He listened as I poured out my pain and confusion. After holding it all in for so long, feeling alone and isolated and insane, like there wasn't one other person in the world who could relate to me, it was a relief to realize that he did.

I know it was his understanding that, for the first time ever, made me feel that I wasn't alone. I wasn't crazy. I wasn't dead. It was a huge relief to know that somebody out there knew exactly what I was dealing with and didn't judge me for it. He didn't reprimand me, didn't hate me, and didn't love me. That was how he got through to me. Despite everything that everyone who loved me had tried to say and do in order to get through to me, nothing had worked before that conversation. And yet there were no profound changes immediately after we talked. There is no miracle cure for anorexia—not even understanding.

He told me to write down his name and number, which I did, and to call him if I ever needed to talk. The conversation ended. I put the phone down. I sat dead still with my broken denial.

Later I trudged downstairs and walked into the kitchen. My mother was there.

"How was it?" she asked. "What did he say?" Her voice was tentative and labored. She anticipated some acknowledgement of my behavior, some awareness in me of the harm I was causing myself.

I lowered my head and sighed. "He is the only person in the world who understands me."

My mother had waited six years for that moment.

Chapter Twelve

CANDYFLIPPING

If I could not escape my mother's pain while living with her, then I would have to escape her altogether.

One month after she threatened to institutionalize me, I left her home and moved to Cape Town to live with my baby sister. I arrived wearing hot pants and high heels while I chain smoked. I looked like a white-trash Barbie doll. My sister had recently discovered Buddhism, so life to her was one infinite chain of perfect synchronicity. I was an uncertified rave bunny, numb, and dead in the head, hopping from one high to the next. We rented a two-bedroom apartment in the city center, for which she paid. Our living room was furnished with hand-me-down wicker furniture from my grandparents' porch. Our bookshelves were lined with empty vodka bottles that we used as candle-sticks. I picked up flyers off the street that advertised raves and trance parties and created a litter collage on the kitchen wall. My sister sat Buddhas on the windowsills and strung Tibetan prayer flags between windows.

My sister's bedroom was near the front door. It was nurturing and warm, a sacred space like an ashram. She draped silk saris over her bed and lit candles and laid down Persian rugs and soft pillows. She had dream catchers and crystals hanging in the windows and had painted the Buddhist mantra for compassion, *Om mani padme hum*, which although almost impossible to translate into English, is often said to mean "praise to the jewel in the lotus," on her wall in Sanskrit. My room was tucked in the back next to the bathroom. It was small and stark and damp like the prison cell floor on which I would soon find myself curled. My window overlooked a tall brick building with rows and rows of tiny windows where people hung their floor mops and laundry out to dry.

My sister shaved her head and wore soft cotton Indian shirts, flowing skirts, beaded leather sandals, and a talisman around her neck. She woke up at sunrise to burn incense and meditate and salute the sun every morning with yoga postures. I used a straightening iron on my bleached hair and wore skin-tight spandex crop tops and fluorescent green Lycra bell-bottoms. I strutted in the door at sunrise after all-night dance parties, wired on ecstasy and shaking, my body torn between exhaustion and adrenaline, fighting sleep.

She lined the kitchen cabinets with jars of lentils and legumes and green tea and prepared chickpeas and brown rice and ate raw vegetables and fruits. I had one tin of cheap instant coffee and a paper bag of refined sugar on the kitchen shelf and empty cigarette packs scattered all over the place. She bought weekly groceries at a vegetable market, spinach and carrots and beets still with their leaves and roots and shoots dangling with gritty soil. I walked to the twenty-four-hour convenience store at the gas station to stock up on a handful of toffee lollipops, which I sucked on all night, every night, as my dinner.

It was summer. There were parties everywhere. Clubs were open till dawn. Teenyboppers partied in the streets. Adults tanned topless on the beaches. Guys got drunk on sex-on-the-beach cocktails at sidewalk cafés, their girls wearing nothing but bikinis and sarongs. Everyone was socializing, serenading, and taking siestas in the sunshine. Basking lazy in the heat like lizards. I spent the days locked up in the apartment drinking whiskey and diet 7UP, eating scraps of food here and there like an insect. I read Irvine Welsh novels with titles like *Ecstasy* and *The Acid House*, identifying with the characters in his books who were unemployed rogues and juvenile junkies in melancholic dead-end towns, doing nothing but getting stoned and drunk and drinking tea in their box homes on gloomy rainy days.

At night I hung out at the bar where my sister worked, thinking I looked mature and ladylike drinking white wine and grenadine with ice, copying some woman I once saw at a bar. Then I went out to party all night at some club or rave. After twelve hours on the dance floor, rushing on ecstasy and speed, I returned home in the morning and prepared myself a bowl, the size of my palm, of baby porridge. On the box was written: "Suitable for infants aged 3–6 months."

I've hardly eaten the whole week. It's Wednesday today. Last week this time I ate a few bites of mozzarella. I've only had some veggies and fruit after that and more pieces of cheese and today a piece of watermelon for breakfast and a bite of fried fish for protein and a teaspoon of barley malt for vitamin B. Will I survive? I'm better than I was mentally. Last week I had halloumi cheese and some tuna salad and a few potato chips. Today I had some broccoli and lentils and so much coffee, sugar, and milk. Yesterday a whiskey and Diet 7UP. Smoking like a chimney.

There is nothing in my head. It's empty. I have independence and free time but I feel guilty for welcoming pleasure. E eliminates this guilt so I can indulge in the pleasure. I'm twenty, going on twenty-one, broke, single, and desperate for true love. I have too much time to think now. I'm so engrossed in myself it's actually boring. Why do I thrive on struggle and suffering? Why do I blame myself so hard? Fuck, I am my own worst nightmare. I should socialize or something. Last night E was terrible. My face is pimply. I feel slow and tired. I've been on such a perpetual hype. I have not stopped. How is it to be back from overseas? I don't think about it. Should I consider a path? I am: beaching, tanning, bumming, drugging, and partying.

My sister tried to inspire me to walk hand in hand with her through her esoteric universe, but I was stuck in my bubblegum world. She ran baths for me and lit candles all around, only I was too suspicious of her kindness. I felt like a homeless girl soaking in my own dirt in a rich lady's spa. While I chain-sucked lollipops and my body feasted on the sugar, my sister prepared fruit and vegetable platters and explained that raw food still contains all its *prana* (life force) and that vegetarianism is part of *ahimsa* (non-violence) to living beings. She played Sanskrit chants in her room and read Hindu scriptures aloud while my house music blasted in the background. When I cried to her that some guy stole my cigarettes at the club, she talked to me about how like attracts like. When she found out I had been stealing for years, she said that bad karma inevitably comes back to you. She then agreed to listen to my stories about it without judging me.

I told her that at my jobs waiting tables at restaurants, instead of handing over the money patrons paid for their dinners, I pocketed most of it. I told her I took fruit from supermarkets and stuffed clothes from clothing stores into my bag. It felt as though taking these things was just a part of me instead of something that was actually immoral, illegal, or a sickness. I felt that it was my right to have these things. I was just taking what was there already. It wasn't something I thought I should give up. Stealing was an adrenaline rush, a high like any other.

The stealing continued compulsively almost as though it had a life of its own. I remained oblivious to the fact that it might have represented a serious mental problem, that kleptomania is not just a euphemism for a petty teenage prank. Even in my first few years of recovery—when I would speak about drug abuse, promiscuity, and cutting—I would not mention the stealing. It wasn't intentional that I left it out. It just didn't seem relevant to anorexia. But I would discover just how relevant it was. I would learn that an anorexic is depriving herself so radically and chronically of food that her restrained energy builds up inside her. This causes an energetic pressure that by its nature has to have some explosive release. I would begin to understand that the drugs, the sex, and the cutting all gave me some sense of release from that pent-up energy. It was the same with the stealing.

One of the tenets of Buddhism is to remain nonjudgmental, so instead of haranguing me like I felt others were doing, or reprimanding me, my sister nudged me, like I was a hatchling with undeveloped wings, standing by my side, believing all along that I would "see the light."

"I read about a woman who claimed not to have had anything to eat or drink in seven years and to have survived only on air," she said. I told her it was bullshit, impossible, and that she should stop reading tabloid magazines, although we both knew I was surviving on cigarette pollution and sugared caffeine.

I bulleted ahead as though I was running on all the fuel in the world. I paid no attention to an old friend who told me that every person tanning on the beach gawked at my bony body in my bikini when I took off my towel. I paid no attention when my sister's friend referred to me as "the sister who lives on an apple a day," nor when she spread it around town as though it were a virus. I paid no attention when I took ecstasy at a club and vomited up black pellets that looked like rat shit or coffee grinds, which years later I discovered was internal bleeding. The only thing I paid attention to was the one and only time my sister lost her cool with me while working two jobs to support us and treating me still like the best friend and beloved sister that she once knew.

My sister really knows how to make me feel shittier than I do already. She said today, "You don't have a job, you don't have any money, you are anorexic—get your act together." I'd never say that to her—it hurts. I'm the black sheep, and I've been sheared to the bone. I don't even care. I have no pity. I want no sympathy. I need no compassion. I hate everybody. E. Only E. Am I this desperate? Do I need to reach the lowest of lows to realize where I am? Sorry to disappoint everybody that I'm not what they expected; maybe I don't want to be. I'm wasting away. I want to just rave, take it up to the highest point and screammmmmmmmmmmmmmmmmmmmmmmmmmmm. Or maybe I just want to be left alone to rot somewhere in a hole.

Sometime after my arrival in Cape Town I must have met up again with my father, who was now living there too, whom I had not seen since he left Israel. I have no recollection of our reunion whatsoever. Nor do I recall when I started answering his calls. I only remember that high on drugs one night, I borrowed his fancy car (and he somehow let me) and because I was paranoid that the police were following me, I reversed to escape the "police" and accidentally crashed his car into a pole so badly that the entire trunk needed to be replaced. I was so high that I thought it was hilarious. And for some incomprehensible reason, although I also thought he would be furious, he was actually far more forgiving than I could ever have anticipated. Maybe it was small acts of forgiveness like these that slowly, slowly made me hate him a little less over time.

Following a night of popping ecstasy and snorting speed, my uncle, my mom's younger brother, asked me to babysit his one-year-old daughter. I arrived at the front door shaking. I folded my arms over my body and pulled my sweater tight around me and tucked my clammy muggy hands into my jeans pockets. My aunt was in the kitchen preparing a quick spaghetti dinner before they went out. Their baby girl was sitting in a high chair with a stained bib around her neck, all five fingers in her mouth as she sucked food off her hand. My aunt tossed olives and cherry tomatoes in the steaming spaghetti and drizzled it with olive oil and fresh herbs and grated parmesan cheese on top.

"Are you hungry?" she asked. "Help yourself. It's not anything special, just a quick and easy meal."

"No, thanks, I've eaten," I lied. The truth was that I hadn't eaten pasta in ages, and olives, olive oil, and parmesan cheese were out of the question.

"Are you sure? Okay, then, would you mind cutting those sandwiches in quarters for her?"

I looked at my baby cousin and her wispy curls and rhubarb cheeks and felt ashamed that my hands were trembling when I patted her head. I thought that in contrast to her innocence, my uncle would see that I was drugged and dirty. I wanted to tell them not to trust me with their daughter. I wanted them to see that I couldn't take care of myself, let alone a baby. I rolled up my long sleeves and cut into quarters the two slices of bread that were squashed together with apricot jam and peanut butter. My cousin grabbed a piece with her dumpy hands and guzzled it down. I felt jealous of her. I hadn't eaten a sandwich in years, and she made it look so easy and effortless. *I am twenty years older than this baby*, I thought, *and yet she eats more in one sitting than I do in a day, more carbs than I've eaten in weeks.* I wiped her hands and mouth with a paper towel and sat down to watch my uncle and aunt eat their casual Italian dinner, wishing that I could be granted permission to do the same.

Once they had finished their dinner, they got up to load

their plates in the dishwasher, grabbed their coats, kissed their baby girl goodbye, thanked me for coming and said they wouldn't be home too late. *Can't they see that I'm unfit for this role? That I'm not to be trusted?* I heard the front door lock shut and turned to face my baby cousin. She reached out her arms for me to lift her out of her high chair. I reached into my back jeans pocket for a cigarette that I would force myself to hold off on smoking until she was in bed.

I had been starving myself on and off for almost seven years, and by that stage, lanugo, the tiny white hairs found on newborns, was growing all over my arms. My chest was so flat it looked as though I'd had a mastectomy. My stomach was concave and hard like a steel soap dish. And every bone in my body pushed hard against my taut skin, making it seem like my joint bones wanted to blast out of their sockets. I was all angles and no shape. All bones and no flesh. I admired the way my hands looked skinny holding a cigarette. The way my wrists looked skinny holding a wine glass. The way my fingers looked skinny stirring coffee. It was as though I was composing still life snapshots of my body parts in my head so as to place myself in some context. Some visual realm. As though if I kept looking at myself at all times, I would somehow keep myself alive. It was not as shallow as vanity. It was a deep obsession with the angles of my bones and the way my limbs moved light in space.

Everything else was confusing. I couldn't piece together anything outside of myself because nothing made any logical sense. When I eventually got a temporary job as a production assistant for party organizers, my task was to run around town depositing checks, picking up supplies, and hoarding receipts. I went about the actions but had no comprehension of why each duty was necessary or what the implications were if I lost receipts or forgot deposits. I did not understand why I was running around with these scraps of paper or what the checks were for or how every facet of the production process would all come together in the end. My mind had undergone a kind of lobotomy that removed my logic and killed my common sense. A part of my mind was missing, switched off—the part that would comprehend my surroundings, gauge reason, provide a framework. The part that told me, *Life is real. This is happening. This is in front of you. This leads to that.* Nothing in my world made any sense. Except piecing together my body. And narrating my life according to the bits and pieces of food I ate over time.

I must confess that I don't know what this shit is about. Every time I eat, no matter what quantity or flavor, I feel sick with guilt. Like I've committed a crime. I feel my thighs swelling and my stomach expanding. I literally struggle to breathe, to inhale or exhale normally. I hyperventilate. I almost never get hungry, and if I do feel it coming, I immediately stop the feeling. I don't know if it's a weight thing or a personality issue. I know I want to be stick thin, but then sometimes I feel too scrawny, but it doesn't make me eat. I want to eat healthy, be healthy, and sometimes I just want to be sick and taken care of, to look waif-like and undernourished and ill. I can't decide why the fuck food is such an issue for me. If I were calorie obsessed, I wouldn't drink alcohol, which I do, and I wouldn't drink milk, which I do. So what's the issue here? I haven't eaten carbohydrates in God knows how long, like pasta, bread, rice, etc., that are banned from my head. Only cereal is a maybe. After my intake of food—be it a bite, a sip, whatever—I grab a cigarette to smoke it down. I always attempt to have a good food day, especially on Mondays or the first day of a new month, but it never works. I am so greedy. So big-eyed. My life is fucked-up. Please, can't I have another one?

One day, I woke up at noon and ran my fingers over the grease on my face and through my straw hair. I kicked the duvet off and lifted my legs onto the adjacent wall and flexed my feet and pointed my toes to see the difference it made to the size of my calves. I rotated my legs so I could see them from all angles and jabbed my thighs and calf muscles with my fingers to see if my flesh wobbled. I made sure that when I tried to pinch the skin over my knees and around my ankles that there was nothing to grip. I pinched so that I could see more bone. I grabbed at the backs of my thighs, pulled the skin back, and squeezed so that my legs looked thinner. Then I brought my legs down and lay on my side and bent my knees so that they were stacked on top of one another. I scrutinized the gap between my thighs, which was the only thing in my life that I allowed to be big. I measured a fist in the gap to make sure that it was not smaller than it was the day before. And for many years, this gap between my thighs was one of the most important things in my life. I did this over and over again and then got up to take a brisk shower.

Before running the water, I climbed onto the edge of the bath and hung onto the shower curtain rail so that I could see my legs and my stomach in the mirror above the basin. I balanced on the ledge, grabbed behind each thigh, and pulled the flesh back to see how big the gap was between my thighs. I stood on my tiptoes and pivoted to the side and then the other side to examine the tone and size of each leg. I smeared the skin over my belly and pulled my non-existent love handles and ran my fingers over my hipbones. I turned to see the line of my ribs on one side and then the other. I wanted to make sure that my stomach was flat as a low-fat cracker. After showering, I grabbed a towel and quickly dried myself off and then got dressed in panties and an undershirt that sagged over my frame. Again I stood on the bath ledge and inspected my body, left and right, up and down, and only then did I start my day.

My day started with a carefully constructed ritual of coffee and cigarettes. And it had to be perfect every single time. I had my special mug, which was long and narrow with a thin rim. It had a picture of cherries on it. I stole it from my ex-boyfriend in Israel—the one who hit me at the beach. I drank my coffee only out of that mug, and nobody else was allowed to touch it. In one sitting I drank three or four cups of coffee, one after the other, and chain-smoked. I boiled the kettle, added hot water to the instant coffee, and then added fat-free milk and five teaspoons of sugar. I measured each ingredient so that it tasted the same every single time. I filled my mug to the brim and carried it out, along with my cigarettes and lighter, onto the Juliet balcony overlooking a mountain that I hardly ever noticed. I sat in a foldout chair, stretched my legs out onto the balcony ledge so I could examine them, and took three sips of my coffee. Then I lit my cigarette and took three puffs. Then three sips of coffee. Then three puffs. Then I stubbed my cigarette out and carried my coffee mug to the kitchen. Boiled the kettle. Added more hot water. More sugar. More milk. More coffee. I sipped it to make sure it tasted exactly the same as before. Then I returned to my place on the balcony and sat down again, stretching my legs onto the ledge and relighting my cigarette. I got up to repeat the whole ritual again and again until an hour had passed and my coffee mug was empty, its ceramic base stained brown and sticky sweet, and I had smoked my fourth cigarette all the way down to the filter.

Without this ritual, I felt incomplete; my day felt wrong and my mind felt out of control. If the phone rang or there was a knock at the door or my sister talked to me and disturbed me, then I stubbed my cigarette out and poured my coffee down the drain and started the whole thing over again because my space had been invaded and my ritual was then soiled. I waited until the disruption passed and I could start again in privacy. This ritual was my substitute for food. Every time my body signaled hunger, I had coffee and a cigarette.

Years later, I learned that my attachment to inanimate objects, like my cherry mug, had less to do with possessiveness and more to do with my need to project my lost sense of self onto objects that would become all-important to me and indistinguishable from my own body. If one of my prized objects broke or got taken away, it was as though a piece of myself was stolen. I screamed at anybody who took one of my cigarettes without asking my permission first, and I carried my pack with me at all times. And I clung to my cherry mug as though it were my only air. The day I dropped my cherry mug and it cracked into pieces was a day I cried for a very long time.

Because of my copious liquid intake and the way I fooled my body into thinking it was thirsty when it was hungry, I developed bladder problems. I ran to the toilet to try to pee a couple of times an hour, at least. I sat on the toilet minutes at a time, pushing pushing pushing, until droplets trickled out of my clogged, bloated bladder. It always felt full, but hardly anything ever came out. I was frustrated that I had this problem, but I made no connection between it and my eating habits. It did not occur to me that my constant urinary tension was a side effect of my starvation strategy, a message from my confused body to drink less coffee and eat more food.

It was the same with my breathing problem. I knew my breathing was strained, particularly when I was about to put food in my mouth, no matter how small the quantity. Every time I was about to eat anything, my shoulders tensed up and my chest closed up and my throat contracted and I felt like I could hardly breathe or swallow. I kept yawning to try and get more air in, but the air was stuck in the ether before I could inhale and jammed inside my throat before I could exhale. I panicked. I yawned. I swallowed. I banged on my chest to let air in and let air out. Nothing. I paced up and down clearing my throat and banging my chest and trying to swallow, trying to breathe. But again, I made no connection between it and my anxiety-provoking eating habits.

I've been to a dietician and a psychologist, but I refuse to help myself. And I know the situation is only getting worse. Each day I promise myself to start afresh. Nothing happens. I don't know what this is all about, but I sure as hell wish I did know. Every time I consume food in whatever quantity, whatever flavor, I feel sick with guilt like I've committed a crime I'm ashamed of, like I must suffer and be punished for it.

Fuck this shit. What is wrong with me? I think it's entirely self-inflicted. It's my own fault. My own choice. But I did not choose to be so fucked-up in this. I hate myself sometimes. I think I've got an excellent figure, but it's still never good enough in my eyes, never toned enough, smooth enough, or thin enough. It's driving me mad. I think I'm losing my mind. And nobody understands. How can they? They think I'm fucked. And every day, I try to start off on a clean slate, to have a "good" day in terms of food consumption. But every day is a failure. I do everything in excess, everything with greed, with "big eyes." I can never do anything in moderation. I can't stop at one cup of coffee and say that was good. I have to have another one straight away. Never one glass. Always two. Never one mouthful. Always two.

I hate it. I feel so guilty. So bad. Fucking hell, it drives me mad. If I were a real anorexic, then I could eat whatever and I wouldn't worry, would I? Maybe I do want to be anorexic, sick, dependent. Why? I don't want to be able to eat whatever I want whenever I want. I need restrictions. I need forbidden things to be denied to me. I feel so unhealthy, so dirty. And every day I wake up and say today will be different, but it hardly ever is. And if it is a success, the next day is back to failure. It's pathetic. I'm embarrassed, but I'm proud. I'm in control—or am I? Who the fuck is this voice inside my head? Telling me you can, you can't. Why can't I just be myself? Who the fuck am I, and what do I want? I really wish I knew. I cannot go on living this way. It's madness, it's stupid, and it's killing everyone around me, and I'm becoming a reclusive bore. My mind is dead. My soul is withering, and my energies are depleted. I can't concentrate on anything else but intake. It's sick. And it's making me mad. I just can't stop.

I can't stop.

Everybody takes one look and says I'm as skinny as a rake, only I can't see it or I don't want to. The thought itself consumes most of my day, the intake, no matter whether it is liquid or fruit or food. It horrifies me, haunts me. I actually cannot breathe with this thought in me. At least I've begun to eat something, a little bit. I've slowly allowed myself—allowed being the operative word—foods I like or presume I like or want / have to / think I ought to like. It's sick. But I've started to eat vegetables, which were previously denied access to my system. I've developed a new love or detest for taste. I can't afford to redevelop these tastes, for I know it will lead me to acceptance—of the food, of the tastes, perhaps invariably and inevitably of myself.

Is this what I'm maybe perhaps truly afraid of: a genuine undiluted pure acceptance of myself? Accept, receive, get, attain, be given, acquire. The opposite of reject, deny, insult, put down. I don't know; it's all too confusing. It's all too sore. My mind is a wash, a turning, turning wash. I'm suffering, but I'm quietly fighting or searching or waiting or setting aside the moment for enlightenment of myself, for that "peace of mind" I've denied myself forever, or for as long as it's been. I want to clear it. I want to be well. It's too sick. But sometimes I eat and I can feel it accumulate in my thighs; it's like a suction; it's an invisible fat bloated ugly leach that appears clinging onto my thighs with every swallow, every grind, every normal function of the digestive system.

I've fucked with this for too long. It's not healthy; it's not normal;

it's sick. But I know the monster is there waiting to pounce on its prey—my flesh and bones, my skin. So I have to carefully contemplate my intake. I have to contrive, deceive my own mind in a conniving way so that my own body is gullible to my mind and my mind becomes the gluttonous pig. Restrictions. Limitations. I need rules. I am vulnerable and weak only to my self-inflicted cruelties, my own masochism, my own torture, for it cannot be inflicted by any other—it is entirely and utterly in my control. Under my command. For I am the only one with access through this oracle. I control what goes in, and I control what goes out. Be it food, words, noises, sound.

What am I saying here? I can't eat; I don't want to eat; I don't want this satisfaction, for it has been a punishment for so long, a sin. I am not ready to reward myself; I am not ready to accept, to forgive, to forget, to confront. I need time to decay the thoughts, to rot the feelings, to starve the mind, to kill the soul. I need to starve; I need to feel hungry; I need to ache. I cannot eat tomorrow; I will starve. This has gone too far. I've tried. I've been eating one small meal a day for the past few weeks. I've looked forward to it each time in a strange sort of way. I can no longer afford this leisure; it's too much too soon. I need to take it easy. To detoxify my body. I don't know what I love or hate anymore. Isn't it what's best for me that I should follow? This is hard for me to accept. I need to condition myself to this way of thinking if I am to defeat my old self.

Who is this new person? Do I know her? Is she the child who was wounded, betrayed, laughed at, mocked, and hurt, who became a vindictive, rebellious, hard, indifferent person? Where has she been hiding for so long? Who has taken care of her? Why is she maybe coming back now? Did I ask for her to return? Where has she been hiding? Is this me talking? I'm definitely not schizophrenic. I don't want a disease, to be labeled anorexic, mad, schizo, psycho. I don't want any labels; I want myself. She was so scared to come out, so scared to get hurt. She's protected herself for so long, covered her vul-

nerability with defenses that even her own mother finds hard to pene-trate. But she is pure and innocent and beautiful and lovely at heart, and she exists because she is strong and so brave and indispensable and ungovernable. I need her back. I need her out to destroy the layers of this rock. I liked her best; she was happy and pure. It's been years. Lost for years. I want to come back. It's me. But I've grown up, and there is no turning back. I can only change what lies ahead. Someday soon.

One night I got dressed to go party at the rave club to celebrate my huge achievement, my hard-earned victory, my long-awaited accomplishment. Earlier that day I had weighed myself. I had finally reached my goal weight. It was the same weight as when I was fourteen and at my lowest weight ever. That night, I wore a black halter top that was cropped like a bra just below my breasts with a thin strip covering the back, skin-tight luminous green Lycra bell-bottoms, and sneakers without socks. My hair was flat-ironed and straight as toothpicks.

For dinner before my all-night dance party, I sliced a tomato in half, broke a carrot in two, and ripped off two pieces of lettuce. I shoved the vegetables in a tiny porcelain bowl used for a Japanese soup starter. This was my meal. After dinner, I dug into my party pack, where I stored drugs that I'd scored. I licked my finger so that the tiny piece of paper soaked in LSD stuck to it, and I placed it carefully on my tongue and sucked on it. Out of the bag I shook a white pill that I would swallow at the club in about an hour so that I would be tripping, hallucinating, dancing, smiling, happy, high, out of my mind, with the universe, everywhere and nowhere, beyond time and space, rushing. This was going to be the night of my life. This was my night to combine acid and ecstasy—this was my night to be candyflipping!

As I walked to the front door to leave the apartment with the acid blot dissolving on my tongue and the ecstasy tablet hidden in my sneaker, I passed by the full-length mirror on the wall near the door. I caught a glimpse of a very thin girl with dead, straight, long, dry, bleached hair and a skimpy outfit like a whorish doll. I turned sideways to look at her. I saw a child. I saw a witch. I saw a dumb blonde. It took a few seconds for my mind to register that the girl in the mirror was me. I looked her up and down.

I was thin, blonde, and tanned, and I was still not happy.

Chapter Thirteen

BAREFOOT IN
THE DAWN

The night that I achieved my goal weight was supposed to be the night of my life, a celebration. But it wasn't. The ecstasy tablet I had taken turned out to be ketamine (a horse tranquilizer sometimes sold as an E substitute in the rave scene), and it made me feel like I was locked inside an airtight jar, floating, dizzy, voiceless, and hallucinating. And after having strived to reach my goal weight and anticipating how happy it would make me feel, once the initial high that I experienced when the number lit up on the scale had died down, I didn't feel any different from before. I realized that I would either need to set a new and lower goal weight or try to maintain the weight I had achieved. I didn't think there could be another option.

A few weeks later, my sister and I were seated in the back of a car hitching a ride with some guys we'd met at the bar where she worked, to an outdoor trance party in an inconspicuous field two hours outside of the city center. Five minutes into the journey, one of the guys offered us acid. I seized the opportunity; my sister declined. He passed a small white piece of paper back

to me, and on it was a flat black dot, slightly bigger than a pinhead, with five pointed corners. I glanced out the window at the
glittering black sky, holding a fallen star in the palm of my
hand.

An hour later, sprawled out in the backseat and giggling
hysterically, I was tripping hard. We veered off the highway and
onto a dirt road that felt like a launching pad and passed a massive power station from outer space until we came to a vast open
field scattered with haystacks that after sunrise would look like
croutons on a bed of lettuce. Eventually our space rocket landed,
and my sister dragged me out onto the long grass. We followed
our hosts, and she looped her arm in mine and led me toward an
intense light beaming down on us. An alien figure loomed behind a massive barricade orchestrating some sort of extrasensory
vibration. My body felt loose and fluid from the acid, and I
wanted to dance. I threw my body around and waved my hands
in the air, grinning like a lunatic.

"Where are we? What is this place?" I asked. My sister
yanked my arm and whispered in my ear. "It's just some guy
with a flashlight standing behind a foldout table collecting
money for the rave," she said. "Calm down, we're just in the
queue!"

The guys paid for us to get in and walked us to a Bedouin-
like chill-out tent and then disappeared for the night. Trance-
heads braided one another's hair and massaged each other's
shoulders and drank *chai* and banged bongo drums. Even though
it was nighttime and we were under a starry sky, there were
fluorescent tubes all around that made everybody's clothes stand
out like bleach stains on black cloth. The more I stared at the
translucent colors, at the swirling circles on the hippies' tie-dye
shirts and the glowing white sheets strewn between branches as
awnings, the more outlandish everyone looked.

Blue alien beings with long noodle-like elastic limbs slinked around a fluorescent totem pole, round and round in never-ending concentric circles, a swirl of bodies stirring a cauldron of light and sound. Thumps, bumps, zaps, pops, whistles, bubbles, prangs, zigzags, whoops, zings, bleeps, plops, doings, clangs, rings, drips, drops, rivets, rockets, tweets, swats, swirls, taps, and blips crept up my spine. My sister and I sat on a pins-and-needles haystack, and I jumped up to flick the hay off me. A massive black tarantula crept over the girl's head who sat right in front of me. I looked around and saw hundreds of upside-down bats that hung from a huge tree. Rats scurried all over the ground, their long tails moving this way and that like tiny windshield wipers. I clutched my sister's arm.

"Where are we? Why are there beasts everywhere? Oh my God, what the hell is this place?"

"I don't know what you are talking about, there is nothing here, I promise, just calm down, don't panic, you've taken some acid, and you're just having a bad trip," she said, leading me away from the noise to a raging bonfire. We sat down on the dirt, and I hugged my arms around my knees. She put her hand on my arm, and I screamed.

"Can't you see them?" I begged. "Maggots! Crawling! They're burrowing into my flesh. They're eating me!"

"Shhhhhhh, calm down. There are no maggots. It's all in your head. It's just your imagination. You are here with me at a trance party. You took some LSD. You're just having a bad trip. Don't panic, okay? The more you panic, the more you will feed the nightmare . . ."

Her voice faded, and my body started slowly to disappear into the ground as though I had sat down in sinking sand. Deeper and deeper it sank as I watched my limbs vanishing like smoke. I gripped my knees tighter and held still as my stomach became a vacuum that sucked my entire being into it. My throat burned raw, and my tongue dissolved. I lost my voice. I could not speak. The music in the distance evaporated, and the voice inside my head, my voice, became an echo. I could not hear. The incandescent strobe lights faded, and everything went black. I could not see. I was without. Within. Somewhere. I was a microdot darting through a black infinite void between intersecting lines of color twisting and contracting and dilating and disappearing like shooting stars. I was a traveling atom speeding through boundless blackness blasting between cotton-thin strobes of light. I was a pinhead ricocheting against dark emptiness and beyond.

It was terrifying to feel nothing at all. To appear not to exist and yet be alive enough to realize it. To be conscious of being but yet not to be myself. To be reduced to everything and nothing all at once. To be gone but yet still be here. Although it had the potential to be the acme of lucidity, the quintessence of consciousness, even in that state there existed the fear that I had forever lost the "I" of my being, my sense of self. Me. After striving for seven long hard years to perfect, tone, thin, and deceive my body, I lost total control over it.

I lost my body.

About eight hours later, I felt something soft near my cheek and warm around my body. I felt myself slowly slip back into my physical being like a confused snake sliding back into its molted skin. I was inside the Bedouin tent, and my sister was sitting behind me with her legs wrapped around me to contain me. She was kissing my cheek, even though her kisses felt inches away from my skin. I was cognizant of touch, of sensation, tingling in my limbs, aching in my belly. My sister lifted me up with both arms and led me slowly out of the tent and away from the party into a field. We stood still, and I heard a faint humming sound far away that was getting closer. My eyes flitted around trying to find a point of focus.

"Come down. Look at me." I heard my sister's voice somewhere far away. "Come down to earth. It's me. Your sister. Can you hear me?"

I listened for her voice and tried to catch it as though it were a passing butterfly, and it slowly lowered me down down down enough to feel my feet on the breathing ground. She helped me unzip my pants and told me to squat and urinate so I could get the acid out of my system. My legs buckled, and she gripped under my arms to keep me up. I saw liquid trickling between my legs but I could not feel it coming out of me. My genitals were numb. My throat dry. My tongue heavy. My eyes strained. My body aching. My jaw locked. My cheeks swollen. My forehead throbbing. My stomach knotted.

Ten hours after I had placed the acid blot on my tongue, the sun began to rise. The party was still happening, and happy hippies threw off their sweatshirts and pranced around the totem pole that now looked like a painted tree trunk in the light of day. Everyone hugged and smiled and caressed and held hands and drank *chai* and still the beat went on and the die-hards pummeled the ground. Warriors. My sister stroked my hair and hugged me. I kicked off my sneakers and dug my toes into the fresh dewy grass. I stood there humbled and liberated. Barefoot in the dawn.

If my sister had not been there with me that night as my guiding light, my guardian angel, I might still be lost out there in the black ether. By the time we arrived back at our apartment, she was depleted. She had a quick shower and crawled into bed and passed out. I, on the other hand, was wide awake, lucid, invigorated. My senses were alert and receptive to light, to warmth, to sound, to colors. My eyes felt wide and clear, and everything was visceral. The furniture shifted like buoys on soft waves. Objects morphed, juxtaposed and multi-layered, a saturation of color and texture and brightness.

I paced the apartment feeling how my joints bent and my body worked, limber and oiled. I felt the morning heat on my skin and a soft breeze blowing my way through the open windows. Every orifice in my body felt open and tingly. I reached for a package of potato chips that someone had left lying around and placed one on my tongue without thinking. My tongue was crawling, and it hurt to swallow. It lolled around, and the chip fizzled and dissolved into an amalgam of flavor. I skipped to the bathroom to take a long shower. I closed my eyes and let the waterfall purify me.

When I got out, before grabbing a towel like I usually did, I stopped to look at my naked body in front of the bathroom mirror. I pushed my face up against the mirror and saw millions of shifting multicolored pixels. I pulled back to see a three-dimensional reflection of my face start to form. I stepped further back to take a look at my whole body. It was the first time ever that I felt gratitude. The first time that I saw myself as I was, without judgment, as I was on a deeper level, inside, my soul in a body. I felt lucky to be me. To be alive. To be allowed to come back into my body after having been so out there the whole night, so out there for so many years. And above all, I felt honored that my soul wanted to return to my body.

Who do I thank for giving me this body? Who do I thank for giving me my self?

For many months my sister had been telling me to "wake up" and to "be conscious," but I had no idea what she meant. Yet once I came down from my acid trip that morning, I suddenly awoke to the world in which my sister had been living. A world filled with love and gratefulness. I realized unexpectedly that a higher power was watching over me and had guided me back into my body, brought me back to life. I felt as though I had died and been resurrected.

My catharsis was, I would come to understand, an out-of-body experience, an astral travel. And the type of acid I swallowed was called a microdot. Albert Hoffman, the Swiss scientist and accidental inventor of this psychotropic hallucinogen known as lysergic acid diethylamide, aka LSD, had dedicated his research to understanding the therapeutic benefits of this mind-altering chemical. Hoffman revered LSD as a "magical elixir" and called it "the medicine for the soul" because of its self-realizing attributes and its ability to awaken the mind to an alternate reality and the soul to consciousness. At the time, however, without knowing any of this, I instinctively regarded my acid trip as a spiritual epiphany. And for the first time in a long time, for a very short while until reality set back in, there was more to life than just the gap between my thighs.

Chapter Fourteen

WILDFIRE

When the sun shines too bright, you seek refuge in the shade. Sometimes the shade is darker than you expected.

Despite my spiritual epiphany, for the next three years, I would make one bad choice after another in a desperate effort to keep my relationship with anorexia alive. It was all I knew. I would take all the negativity that anorexia fed on to the extreme. My awakening would not put a stop to the chain reaction that had been building over the years. When you are on the brink of losing someone you are inextricably attached to, no matter how destructive the bond, you will do whatever it takes to hold on no matter what the cost to you. And when you are trapped in an abusive relationship with yourself, it makes it that much harder to walk away.

My choice in men in my early twenties proved as noxious as the drugs I ingested and as empty as the calories I consumed. I was attracted to men who sniffed out my desperation like police dogs, and I found myself embedded in fast flings that inevitably crashed. Just after my sister's words about how like attracts like, I started seeing a guy I was raving with at the time. He had wildcat eyes and a possum-tail ponytail, and he wore unbuttoned Hawaiian shirts that showed off his six-pack abs and tight surfer shorts. I was enamored of his voice because he swallowed his words and clenched his teeth when he spoke, which made it sound muffled in an exotic way.

I found out later that he had the standard voice of crack addicts and that he was a lying, cheating kleptomaniac. All he wanted was my roof over his head for the summer. He was everything I needed to keep me feeling the familiarity of an unloving bond. He was everything I thought a guy should be—an asshole taking his chances on a dumb broad. One night at the club, after he spat cuss words in my face to make sure I knew he was dumping me, I ran home in tears. When I opened the front door and saw that all his things were gone, I realized he had found another place to stay.

If the men I attracted along the way refused to hold my hand or tell me that I was beautiful, the drugs would be there to make me feel like the belle of the ball and to hold my hand all night and not let go till morning light. There was a different drug for every occasion. Ecstasy was my first and best friend for a while. It took some time to warm up, but once it did, it knew how to make me feel like the happiest person alive. It gave me love and showed me how to love. On the first night we met, it wrapped me up in a warm tingly glow of infinite pleasure that I had never felt before and would never feel again. But in time, it would let me down, not show up, and lose interest in trying to make me feel good.

Acid was the stimulating companion with whom I had the most intense connection, so much so that I limited my time with it and saved it for special occasions. Marijuana was a casual friend that failed to stimulate me; whenever we met, I felt paranoid and ill at ease. I tried to avoid it. Heroin was a one-night stand. It confused me. First it made me sick until I vomited, and then it floated me onto a cloud until finally it made me more paranoid than marijuana. From then on I avoided it. Cocaine was my favorite friend. It annihilated my appetite completely and allowed me to drink half a bottle of whiskey without getting so much as tipsy. As long as I paid it ongoing attention, it entertained me the whole night. It lifted me up immediately, stimulated my thoughts, and set them racing in every direction. It made me feel powerful and charged, like a secret agent on a mission that nobody else knew about. But it was my five-day affair with diet pills that finally got me in real trouble.

It was around the New Year when I hung out dancing at the club night after night with my diet pills. The more I swallowed, the faster and longer I danced. One night I danced at the club for twelve consecutive hours, and when the club emptied and the music stopped and the brooms came out to sweep the plastic litter and the fluorescent bulbs switched off and the psychedelic patterns looked like children's squiggles and the chill-out zone was thick with cigarette butts and stained sofas, I could not stop dancing. My body was in cruise control, and anorexia was in love.

For five days in a row I ate nothing but diet pills and did nothing but tan on the beach and rave at the club. The side effect of the pills—other than complete lack of appetite—was that I could not sleep at all. I remember adding up twenty-four plus twenty-four plus twenty-four plus twenty-four plus twenty-four equals 120 hours sleep-free. I was proud of my one-woman marathon. *I can survive on no food and no sleep forever*, I thought. I was able to defy my needs, and that made me superhuman. Invincible. On the fifth night, I caught a ride to the club with a guy I'd met the night before. On the way there, he pulled over in a dingy part of town to score cocaine from a drug dealer's house, a dealer who I found out later was number one on the police hit list. After paying for it at the door, he climbed back into the car to cut a line on a CD cover. That's when I heard police sirens and a flashlight blinded my eyes.

"Where the fuck do I hide this?" the guy screamed. Before I could respond, he threw the folded piece of paper—the size of a matchbox—containing the cocaine, in my lap. Police hands slammed against my window.

"Get out of the car. You are under arrest!" I grabbed the tiny envelope and shoved it down the front of my bikini bottom that I had not taken off for five days and covered my bikini again with my loose bell-bottom sweatpants. The door opened, and two hairy arms pulled me out of the vehicle and shoved me in a police van between two huge uniformed men with guns on their hips and mockery on their tongues. They talked over me like I was some kind of foul smell.

"Put your hands on your knees. Keep them there. Don't move. Just wait till you get to prison, girl, you will love it there."

There, a rubber-gloved policewoman stripped me down to do a full-body search. She swiped my armpits, under my flat breasts, between my legs, front and back, and found nothing. I prayed that the cocaine had gotten lost somewhere along the way. But then I slipped off my sneakers and pulled off my socks, and we found the tiny envelope. It had fallen down from my crotch, through my loose bikini bottom, down my bell-bottom sweatpants, and into my baggy sock. She tasted it and laughed. She called other police in to taste it, and they laughed. I was shoved in a holding cell. I sat on a steel chair under bright lights. My sneaker laces and luminous bracelets and glasses were confiscated.

"Your mother is going to find out about you," said the police officer in charge.

He stared at my hard stomach and my belly ring with a luminous green cross dangling off it. My tiny shirt covered only
my bikini top, and my bell-bottom sweatpants fell down at my
waist, exposing my bikini bottom's drawstrings.

"If I had a daughter like you, I would lock her up too," he
said. "Mark my words, your mother will find out about what a
little bitch you are."

I wished his words could escape me the way the white envelope that fell down my leg had, but they frightened the hell out
of me instead.

"You get to make one phone call," he barked. "Make it
quick."

I called my sister, who was at a twenty-first birthday party,
drunk. It was the early hours of the morning, but she came over
immediately and brought along my wallet and ID, which I had
left at home, as well as my address book.

"This is your one chance to call a lawyer to get you out of
this shit," the police officer said.

I turned to my sister. "Fuck! Who are we going to call? The
only lawyers we know are Daddy's friends, and he's always said
he'd kill any motherfucker who gives us drugs," I whispered.

"And Mommy's friends would tell her for sure—and knowing her, she'd be on the next plane here and would want to
spend the night with you in your cell," said my sister, rummaging
through my address book for contacts. "Hey, what about that
guy you met at my bar a couple of weeks ago? Remember? The
one you went partying with that night. Wasn't he a lawyer?" she
said.

"Shit. He even gave me his business card. I'm sure I kept it
because it was so cool," I said, grabbing the address book out of
her hands and fingering through it. "Here it is! I knew I kept it."
I flashed the yellow card at her. It had his name and number on

the front, and on the back was an image of jail bars, below which it read: *Chance. Get-out-of-jail card—This card may be kept until needed or sold.*

I needed it. "Hey," I said to the police officer through the holding cell's bars. "I know who to call."

"Better make it quick," he snapped. "I got no time for bullshit."

I hesitated before calling the number on the card, but I had no choice. A groggy voice answered. I apologized for calling so early in the morning, and I explained who I was.

"Jesus, it's about two in the morning. What are you doing waking a guy up so early?"

"I got arrested," I said, "And they're making me spend the night in jail unless you can bail me out."

He burst out laughing after I told him why I was arrested. "How much money have you got on you?" he asked.

I heard him fumbling around for something. "None," I said.

"Well, then you're going to have to spend the night there. It'd cost approximately three thousand to get you out now. Or three hundred if you wait until morning."

"Fine, I'll wait."

"You're a fucking lucky girl," he said. "Today's a public holiday, and it's my day off. Next time you want to snort coke in a car, try to be discreet about it, okay? That way you'll avoid getting caught. And you'll be letting a tired man get his beauty sleep."

"Okay. Thanks," I said. "I don't know what I'd do without you."

The officer grabbed the phone out of my hand and ordered my sister to leave. He locked me alone inside a dimly lit cell. It had dirty cement walls with graffiti that read *fuck the prosecutor* and *this is a hellhole* and *I hate you and you will never get out of here.* The roof was chicken wire, and I could see the black sky.

There was a shit-stained steel toilet in one corner and a dirty gray blanket folded in another. With no stimulants and no distractions, I was forced to slow down. But my head was still so intoxicated that I couldn't comprehend that there would be consequences to my arrest. With nowhere to run, I felt contained. I crawled onto the blanket and fell asleep for the first time in five days. Later that morning, I woke up with the sun, rolled my pants up to my knees, and basked in the heat, as though I were on some paradise beach, and I waited for the lawyer to come rescue me.

That afternoon, I appeared in court to stand trial for possession of cocaine. My sister had brought money she earned from waiting tables to pay my bail. My lawyer donned his black robe and put on his highfalutin advocate voice to plead my innocence before the judge. A couple of nights later, he would disrobe and put on the sly voice of a guilty man hiding too many secrets. And I quickly discovered, while he wined me and dined me on sashimi and whiskey on the rocks, that this thirty-two-year-old man was a veteran cocaine and heroin junkie. We laughed about our affair being founded on the irony that the night we originally met at my sister's bar, a couple of weeks before, he had taken me under his wing and introduced me to cocaine, which I snorted off a toilet seat cover through a rolled-up bill plugged into my nostril. And within a week of the trial, I was practically living with him. My lawyer. My drug lord. My sugar daddy.

The next time he defended me in court—for the same incident—after a late night of drinking whiskey like water and snorting railway lines of cocaine going nowhere, we both showed up sleep deprived and wired, reeking of booze. After court was adjourned, and my case postponed, we drove around the city in his beat-up car smoking cigarettes and pumping trance music through the speakers. He pulled over on the roadside, kissed me, and slipped a tiny white envelope into my jeans pocket. He balanced the trance CD cover carefully on the hand brake. I emptied the white powder onto the iridescent sparks shooting out of the black hole on the plastic CD cover as he used his credit card to chop perfect white lines with the finesse of a fine chef.

I remember thinking that if I could do cocaine for the rest of my life, I would be the happiest person in the world. It felt like a blessing to have reached my twenties and to be able to make that choice, which seemed such an adult one. I believed that if I did cocaine often enough, I could avoid the comedown, and the happy high would last a lifetime. But the high lasted until the end of the CD and happiness until the last line.

My sugar daddy was squatting in a dark derelict house overlooking an alley, with iron bars on the windows and curtains drawn to shut out the sun. A huge black plastic trash bag full of marijuana was stuffed behind the refrigerator, and he hauled it out, every other day, to ration some out to his regular customers. The lounge had a torn sofa and a TV with bad reception; his bedroom had a mattress on the floor, and his clothes hung on a thin pole rack. The spare room had an octagonal poker table, where his crusty cocaine cronies came over every other night to practice their straight faces and fibs. I strolled in wearing denim shorts and a toddler-size tank top with a Superman logo, cocktail waitressing for the night, and sat on my sugar daddy's lap to snort white powder off the broken mirror that was passed around.

My sugar daddy offered me exactly the lifestyle that I craved to keep my self-destruction going. All I needed to do was keep up with him and play the part. In the three years that we were a couple, I only remember him asking me about my eating once. We had been together for one week, and he suddenly noticed that food was not part of my daily routine.

"Do you have an eating disorder?" he asked.

"Why do you ask?" I was surprised that he noticed.

"Just asking. I haven't really seen you eat much."

He is so observant, I thought. The fact that he cared enough to say something made me feel acknowledged, which quickly led me to believe it was true love.

A couple of weeks later, he broke the news to me that he had applied for another job in another city and had been accepted for the position. He would be handing my case over to his father, the best criminal lawyer in Cape Town. He would be packing everything up and leaving within a few weeks. He would be moving to the right-wing, racist, conservative city of Pretoria, an hour away from my hometown of Johannesburg. He made it clear that he did not think it would be a good idea for me to follow him and said he would visit every month. He admitted that he would prefer sporadic flings over a live-in relationship. Before his departure, he organized a job for me waiting tables at a greasy steak house owned by a 'friend' of his. I later discovered this owner was the most notorious cocaine dealer in Cape Town, who hired only female staff willing to wear mini skirts and fake smiles. After my sugar daddy left, he visited me about one weekend a month for one year. I was still living with my sister the whole time in our city apartment and working at the depraved steakhouse or some other place. I was so negligent as a waiter that each meager restaurant job bled into the next, I barely remember them all, let alone each derelict one distinctly.

After a year of agonizing over when my sugar daddy would next surprise me with monthly visits of weekend binges, I wanted more—more from him and more from the drugs. I was free to leave Cape Town because, thanks to his father's legal expertise, my court case was eventually dropped, and I was acquitted. By that time I had ashamedly confessed to both my parents all about my arrest and trial and they were both incredibly supportive. I had been so scared to tell my father that I asked my uncle, my mom's brother, to accompany me to break the news because my father had always said he would literally kill anyone who offered my sister and me drugs. So I made the decision to move to Pretoria to live with my sugar daddy, even though he still didn't think it was a good idea. What I didn't know was that I would be getting a depressant for a partner who drowned his woes in weekend heroin binges and went cold turkey during the week. Meanwhile, as long as we were in it together, as long as there were parties to attend, drugs to do, and fun to be had, our relationship worked. His drug addiction and my food addiction were in cahoots with each other on a mission to negate as much of our past and present as we could, with the unspoken understanding that neither of us would question the other about our addictions.

We moved into a triple-decker condo with painted walls the color of urine, a dead vegetable garden, and a glass liquor cabinet. Later we found out that it used to be a gay brothel. In bed at night, my sugar daddy told me that he could still smell stale man sex in the room. On weekends, we lay in bed compiling grocery lists of recreational chemicals for the following night's party: acid, ecstasy, magic mushrooms, coke, weed. On weekdays, my depressed new "hubby" returned home in a worn-out suit, hit the bottle, and hugged the TV, and together we polished off thick red wine and planned our weekend agendas.

I went through stages of bingeing on pots of spaghetti Bolognese and cheap Chinese takeout, but for the most part I had one standard routine: complete calculated control. I ate nothing for breakfast. Throughout the day, I ate a bunch of bananas, including the bitter pith inside the peel, which I grated with my teeth until I tasted rubber and digested every single long string. Come evening every day, I swam one hundred lengths in the pool at the gym, not a length more, not a length less, and then did an hour of weight lifting. Or I drove an hour each way to Johannesburg to do my Fatburn aerobics class. When I got home, I opened a bottle of wine and prepared a dinner of lettuce leaves and thin slices of low-fat cheese, and then I started it all over again the next day.

Drugs and alcohol got me through the night and helped me party until sunrise, but I needed something to get me through the days, to occupy me in the downtime and to keep me active when clubs were closed or aerobics classes were over. The work I had found at restaurants and bars over the years actually supported my lifestyle and matched the cardiovascular workout I got from dancing and exercising. One would think it ironic for an anorexic to choose waiting tables as a full-time occupation, but it was perfect. Waiting tables involves tasks that are repetitive, regimented, and mindless, which stops overanalyzing and obsessing. The work was a tainted form of meditation for me because although I was confronted all day long with food, thoughts about my personal consumption were obliterated. I raced around memorizing orders, pushing production, small-talking, and serving customers' unrelenting carnal needs all day and those of hungry drunk perverts all night. There was never a second to think about my own needs. Managers were always on the lookout for waitresses desperate for something—be it money or a respite from their minds. Their businesses depended on waitresses working double shifts.

And so, after living for a few months in Pretoria, I found a job waiting tables at a busy restaurant seven days a week. My weekend shift started at 7:00 a.m. on Friday. On our fifteen-minute break at 10:00 a.m., the other waiters ordered bacon and eggs, French toast and omelets. I ordered two slices of thin toast with butter. On our half-hour break at 4:00 p.m., the other waiters ordered barbecued chicken, hamburgers, and French fries. I ordered three side orders of spinach. Then I was back on my feet, pushing through the night downing diet sodas laced with alcohol until 3:00 a.m. on Saturday, when I would drive home drunk, skipping all the red lights.

For twenty non-stop hours, I served a raucous crowd of unhappily married suits that arrived in droves with their week's worth of pent-up aggression and their life's worth of demands. They were all bald, ugly, pot-bellied, middle-aged men who were there to get as pissed as their pockets would allow and to bet their sick luck on waitresses whose sole aim was to get them to order more booze and therefore increase their tips at the end of the night. I skirted around tables and chairs, bombarded by the perverted murmurs of drunken men. One morning, I sidled up to a boozed-out old sod who brought his wife and kids in for brunch on Sundays, and I offered him another drink. He grabbed my waist and slipped his hand down to pat my ass and rested it there, and I let him because I wanted his money.

For those twenty hours, I was forbidden to lean against a wall, a counter, the bar, or even near the kitchen behind the waiters' station. I was fined every time the manager caught me leaning. Sometimes, after midnight, I snuck behind the waiters' station and crouched down from exhaustion, sick from all the booze I stole off the tables and the lack of food in my stomach and the insane hours. But the manager always found me and told me to get back on my feet and get out there—to put on a happy face and serve my customers. It was voluntary slavery. And I could not do without it. Hard work was the fuel that kept me going. As long as I worked hard, I escaped myself. And as long as I escaped myself, I made it through the day. On the rare occasion that I wasn't allocated a shift, I begged another waiter to let me cover his or her shift so I wouldn't have to spend one minute alone.

After a year, however, I was fired. Even though I was secretly sick of working there, I would never have admitted it because it was my salvation. But firing me that day was like confiscating my drug. Permanently. It was forcing me to go cold turkey. The manager called me into his office to tell me he was tired of getting complaints from customers about my service and that it was time to let me go. In protest, I screamed at him, kicked his chair, and told him he had no right to betray me and that I would take him to court for unfair dismissal. He stared at me with blank eyes and told me to leave.

I stormed out, tore off my apron, marched to the restroom, slammed the door behind me, crouched down, held my gut, and cried silently. When I heard knocking on the door, I pulled myself up off the floor and punched the wall and slammed the door behind me and stomped out. The entire restaurant stared at me. I didn't care. I passed the table that got me fired, and I wanted to spit in their faces and swear out loud. But I didn't. I controlled my rage and hissed vile words under my breath. And all the anger that I felt at the world and at managers who had molested me and fired me and at men who had used me and abused me accumulated in that moment, and I wanted to explode. I wanted to destroy and hurt and beat and punch and kick—but the only way that I knew how to cope with such emotions was to internalize them. So that is what I did. I took all that immense, burning build-up of insurmountable fury, and I internalized it.

I starved another day.

———

Two years of living a risqué and debauched lifestyle in Pretoria with my sugar daddy were enough to taint our romance and kill the novelty of the drugs. Besides, the latter had ceased to work the way they used to. Having cocaine freely available every night of the week dulled the ritual to routine. The highs wore low, and each comedown left me with clammier hands, colder sweats, and a deeper emptiness than the one before. I also became intolerant to ecstasy, which either made me throw up or had no effect at all, and I started having one bad acid trip after another. Plus, starving, overexercising, and overworking were no longer enticing enough. I needed something else or someone else to keep me alive. I was bored with waking up to an older man who slumped out of bed every morning and asked me which tie he should wear to the office. And together, we were bored with our daily drudgery of drugs and drinking. I wanted more fun, more escape, and more kicks, because if I stopped the adrenaline rush, I would be forced to slow down and face a frightening and unfamiliar reality.

Paradoxically, however, since my spiritual epiphany three years earlier, there had been the slightest, subtlest faith germinating inside me. I was slowly becoming aware that I was a spiritual being leading a physical existence. I took my belly ring out because somebody told me it drained the life force from my solar plexus, which I learned was my third chakra. I bought a hand-made eco-friendly journal and confided in it my spontaneous realizations of a higher meaning. I wanted so much to share my new journey with somebody. But my sugar daddy was not interested; he was all too set on corroding his already-blackened soul. So it would not be long before I left him behind to dig his own grave.

That summer, before I broke up with my sugar daddy, I flew to Cape Town to visit my sister and my mother who had recently left her home in Johannesburg and had relocated there. There was a photography show open to the public where photographs could be submitted and hung anywhere from street corners to restaurant walls. My mother had encouraged me to partner with a young photographer she knew so we entered together and were accepted. It was there, in Cape Town, that I found my scapegoat. He was a six-foot-three Dutch model with thick blonde spiky hair, Japanese eyes, caramel skin, and a deep seductive voice, a suave hunk who made every woman in town stick to him like resin. And if he wanted me, even if he would sometimes make me sleep on the floor because he said he needed his space, even if he would sometimes seduce men behind my back or tell me he was still deeply in love with his ex-girlfriend, it still meant I was worthy. Of his "hotness," at least.

He owned a tapas bar in town called Diablo—Spanish for *devil*—which was where the young photographer, his friend, had chosen to hang our photographs. We met for the first time and instantly connected across a crowded room. Love at first sight. We were both lost souls in search of higher meaning, mine as silent as his was salient. Together we seized the nightlife with a devil-may-care attitude. We were soul mates. Blood siblings. We slept all day and talked all night about esoteric topics like universal synchronicity, and we read aloud to each other from books with titles like *Conversations with God*. He taught me to close my eyes, focus on my third eye, and meditate. He showed me how to greet him with *namaste*—which means, "I salute the divine within you." We marveled at our unfathomable instantaneous bond. I felt I had finally found my other half and thought he did too. He was my prince in black leather pants who had come to rescue me from my crumbling castle.

One night, after he had closed the restaurant, we locked the door and got so wasted on a bottle of tequila that we ended up having sex on the cement seating visible to the street while a gang of street kids ogled at us through the glass door. I was so drunk that I only came to mid act only to realize what had happened. I knew then that it was over with my sugar daddy. I had betrayed him and there was no turning back. This drunken act was my way out. I soon after returned to Pretoria to break up with my sugar daddy, pack up my belongings, and relocate to Cape Town.

Months later, once I was living in Cape Town, my prince and I both worked nights, the prince at his tapas bar and me right next door as a bartender at Cape Town's hotspot bar of the season. After work, in the early hours of the morning, we turned the music up and danced on his or my bar counter, and then we paraded our scantily dressed selves around town, wasted on gold tequila that we downed with hot chilies. We danced in the streets in the pouring rain and smoked on sidewalks, dangling our long legs above the gutters. We were small-town amateur exhibitionists with big egos, Bonnie and Clyde. During our free time, we rode his Vespa on highways, me facing backward, free spirits on a wild ride, along windy roads giving the fuck-you finger to passersby. We paraded our sunburned bodies on scorching beaches, him in purple velvet underpants and me stark naked except for a transparent black G-string. One morning, after a sleepless night where we polished off a bottle of tequila on empty stomachs, we popped five ecstasy tablets each—that was the very last time I ever did E—and rode on his Vespa to a deserted beach; drunk, dehydrated, and deliriously happy, we believed we were in love and invincible.

And maybe we were at the time, but the prince and I lived in secrecy like city rats in his basement apartment that we painted in dark colors with coarse outdoor cement paint. We went without baths or showers for days because neither of us bothered to wash. There was a dirty futon on the ground and an empty clothes cupboard because our clothes covered the floor like a tattered rug. The kitchen was infested. Trash bags would sit inside stinking because neither of us threw them out. Ants and cockroaches crawled all over rotting avocado skins that were left on the kitchen counter, and flies nestled in the empty tomato-juice cans. Although I nibbled on the occasional avocado or tapas at his bar, for the most part I ate nothing but a mango a day with tiny pieces of pale cheese that would barely lure a mouse to a trap. Alone in his basement apartment, I climbed, with my meals, behind the bars in the windows and sat on a small ledge overlooking an empty lot and bird shit. This was my private ritual that preceded my bar shift night after night.

At job after job, I had worked myself to the bone, but my bartending stint at the hotspot bar would be the last of its kind, where I would work twelve-hour shifts, from 5:00 p.m. till 5:00 a.m., dressed in skimpy tops that exposed my iron belly and tight pants that hugged my bony ass, serving hard liquor to hardcore drunks who leched after the G-string sticking out of my pants. Same old story. I had streaked my hair with peroxide and poured red henna over it so it glowed like fire—long bright orange-red-yellow glowing streaks. It graced my back like a flaming mane, ablaze. My energy screamed; *I* was on fire, burning. I drank leftover margaritas and pink daiquiris and any other cocktail that I had concocted, and I slammed tequila shots on an empty stomach. Sometimes, when I poured shots for customers, I turned my back on the crowd and poured one for myself. Like I owned the place. Not for one minute did I think that I didn't.

There were nights I blacked out completely from the alcohol. There were nights I didn't black out but just didn't sleep. There were nights I slammed so many tequilas that after work I curled up and passed out on the bar counter until morning.

There were nights I vomited in the bar's toilet, blacked out, and woke up with my drunken skull rested on my arms on the toilet seat, my legs wrapped around the toilet bowl like a spent serpent. I sat there on the filthy floor, too tired and too wasted to stand up. It was my final purge. I would later be told by my nutritionist that, ironically, it was the drinking that saved my life. She said that the sugar in the alcohol supplied what my body lacked and kept me going. Only I was going nowhere.

One night, the police raided the bar. They charged in, and I turned the music up full blast and played Placebo's notorious track about heroin addiction from the album *Without You I'm Nothing*. The song explained exactly what my life was like. Anorexia was my lifeblood. Without my thin, perfected, anorexic image, my cold dead numbness, I felt I was nothing. But in truth, all that was left was a tortured self, a precarious persona. A fake me.

For a few more weeks I raged ahead like wildfire; then I burnt out.

Chapter Fifteen

SURRENDER

Summer died. The green leaves dried brown. The barflies went back to their day jobs. The tourists migrated north. It was then that I returned to Pretoria to break up with my sugar daddy and pack up all that was left of my life there so I could relocate to Cape Town to be with the prince and start over, again.

I had left my most personal belongings scattered around the spare room. My sugar daddy was at work that morning, and I sat alone in an ugly silence on a cold tiled floor sifting through boxes bloated with memories. Outside the barred windows, the wind whistled a lonely lull, and the dry sky faded dim. The horizon was a murky ginger thread. And up my spine crept a shadow. I rolled up the sleeves of my faded gray sweatshirt and ran my hand through my charred hair. The henna had washed out, and all that was left was dead bleached strands. The makeup had rubbed off, the fancy dress was torn, the costume party was over. I felt a dull heat in my chest, and my eyes stung. I hunched my back and hugged my legs to my chest and lay my head on my knees.

When I looked up again, the shadows in the room were

contrasted by a bluish twilight. I got up and paced back and forth, taping up boxes and stacking them, sifting through papers and tossing them or piling them. I went through pile after pile of papers, crumpling up one page after another. Then, hours later, I came across a small, faded yellow piece of paper with Rob's name and number—the man who had spoken to me over the phone about my eating disorder when I retuned home from the army. The man who had managed to break through my denial.

I had hidden it in the hope of forgetting his words, just as I had hidden my anorexia, hoping to forget it too. I remembered that he had said that I should keep in touch and let him know how I was doing and that I should always feel free to call him whenever I wanted, even if it was just to say hello. I didn't think he would remember me if I called. But I folded the paper with his information quickly anyway and stuffed it in my jeans pocket and taped up the last of the boxes. Somewhere in my thawing heart, I must have known it was a sign, because a couple of days later, before leaving Pretoria behind, I felt compelled to call him.

"Of course I remember you!" he said. "How the hell are you?"

"Fine."

"What's it been, like, three or four years since I talked to you?"

"Something like that."

"Wow, time flies, hey, girlie? Where are you?"

I told him that I had only just found his number and that I was in Pretoria.

"Great, then you are in my neck of the woods," he said, even though he lived an hour away.

I told him that I wasn't staying, that I was leaving for Cape Town in a few days.

"What's waiting for you in Cape Town?" he asked. I didn't
have an answer. "I'll make a bargain with you, girlie: you visit
me and say hello, I wish you well on your journey, and off you
go. How does that sound?"

I hesitated.

"Have we got ourselves a deal?"

I said that maybe I could drop by after class the following
night, which was in Johannesburg anyway.

"Great. You see, now there's a plan. What are you studying
nowadays?"

"Nothing. It's an aerobics class," I said.

There was silence on the other end. "Okay!" he said cheer-
fully, interrupting the silence.

"Now don't forget to swing by. I'll be expecting you." We
said goodbye; I put down the phone and sensed a spasm in my
chest, like a deep sigh wanting release.

I don't know why I went. Part of me wanted to prove to
him that I had changed. That I was now grown up. Mature. Independent. Well. Part of me wanted affirmation. Confirmation.
His stamp. *This one is good to go. This one has a destination. This
one is on the right road. Getting there. Doing it. A role model.* Or
maybe I really wanted someone to see through me. To see my
disguise. To notice my vulnerability. To listen to the little girl
inside who was screaming for help but thought that nobody
could hear her.

On a Tuesday night after my aerobics class, I showered and
got dressed in my baggy gray sweatshirt and black sweatpants
and tied my wet hair back tight in a long ponytail. *I will prove to
him that I am fine*, I thought. *I will go there, and he will put his
hands on my shoulders and look at me and smile. You're all right,
girl, he will say, you're doing just fine. I will have his blessing and
his backing. I will be just fine.*

It was dark when I found his house. An old dark blue car was parked in the driveway. A dim light shone onto stone paving. I had called him from my cell phone on the road to ask for directions again. And then I called him again to tell him I was lost. And then again to tell him I still couldn't find the house. Finally, I parked on the opposite side of the street, pulled up the hand break, and clutched the steering wheel with both hands. I slicked back my hair, pulled my sleeves further down over my fingers, and cinched the drawstring of my sweatpants tighter around my waist. I got out of the car ready to lie.

I crossed the street, and a stocky man with bulbous calves and a balding head stood in the driveway to usher me in. He wore navy blue canvas shorts and old flip-flops and a white collared T-shirt. He had gold-framed square glasses and spoke even louder than he did on the phone. He thrust his hand out to shake mine and told me to come on in. *I have made a huge mistake coming here*, I thought. *This man is not what I expected him to be. What was I thinking?*

Four hours later, however, I was still talking with him, even though he did most of the talking. He knew that I had arrived wearing my unconvincing attitude of "I'm fine." And the more I insisted that I was fine, the more he told me that I wasn't. He told me that he dedicates his life to helping girls recover from eating disorders and educating them and their families. He talked about his book on eating disorders and about the ability of the disorder to do irreparable damage to the body and the mind. His face softened and his voice quieted down when he told me about his daughters' sicknesses and recoveries, about some girls who died and others who made it.

"This is not a game, my girl," he said. "You are playing with your life. Do you get that? This is your life, and you only get this one shot at it."

He said I would need to break the cycle of the dysfunctional family by fully recovering from anorexia so that my children wouldn't suffer the same pattern. And lastly he said, "Only once you are fully recovered will you meet the man who will be your life partner."

"I've got someone already," I said, thinking of my prince.

"Well, he ain't gonna be the one," he said.

"How can you say that?"

He crossed his arms, shook his head, and pursed his lips. "Sorry to have to break the news to you, but there is absolutely no way in hell that you can live your life with someone if you can't yet live it on your own."

He uncrossed his arms and his legs, stood up, pushed his chair back, and stretched.

"Now you best be on your way, kiddo. It's gettin' late, and you've still got a long way to go." He hugged me like I was a cuddly doll and slapped me on the back. "But before you leave," he said, "I have something for you."

He handed me a book he had written, titled *The Unknown World Behind Eating Disorders*. On the back cover was the word *happiness* written in bold above a tiny picture of a bird with open wings soaring above the whole round ball of Earth. Below it the words of William James read: "The greatest revolution of our generation is the discovery that human beings, by changing the inner attitudes of their minds, can change the outer aspects of their lives."

I opened the book to a random page. An excerpt read: "It will take approximately five years to recover from full-blown anorexia."

"Five years?" I gasped.

Rob looked at the page and said, "At least. What are you now, early twenties? Then you'd better get started on your five-year plan, don't cha think? Here, take this with you."

He held out a small square piece of paper with a name and number on it.

"I want you to promise me that as soon as you get to Cape Town, you will make this one call, if that's the only thing you do."

I took the piece of paper from his hand and scanned it.

"It's the name and number of an excellent psychologist in Cape Town who runs a support group for girls with anorexia and bulimia," he said.

I knew I felt tired of being on the run. Tired of being a convict on the loose. By taking the piece of paper, I was handing myself in. I was admitting to my guilt. Why would felons allow themselves to get caught if not to end their chase?

"I want you to take it only if you promise to make just this one call. That is all you have to do for now, girlie."

I said I would. I knew I wanted to speak out. I knew I wanted to say something. I knew I wanted to meet other people like me. I knew I did not want to suffer alone anymore. And I knew that as much as I had tried to convince myself otherwise, I was still fucked-up. And I did not know how to get out, even though I had tried for so many years on my own to eat properly. I knew that reaching out for support could help, but I didn't know that it could also hurt worse than anything I had ever felt before.

The night before my departure, I headed out on the lonely, liberating highway across cities for my last aerobics class, after which I went to the gym's sauna. That night, there was nobody else inside. I spread my towel out, lay down, breathed deeply, and felt rejuvenated and yet exhausted. My head was empty and clear. I lay there in the intense heat completely still, listening to my heartbeat.

Why do I turn to food? Why do I starve myself? Why do I diet so obsessively?

There was something about the solitude and heat and relaxation of that moment that put me in the right space to receive an answer. I realized that my anorexic state was also a spiritual state. When my mind was confused and my emotions felt heavy, I starved my body in order to feel lighter inside because I had begun to believe that I was mind, body, and soul.

Making my body physically lighter, thinner, is an attempt to compensate for my heavy emotions.

The realization itself made me feel emotionally lighter because it occurred to me that there had to be more to my anorexia than what I understood. I knew that if it was spiritually related, then maybe I would eventually find meaning in it.

Upon my arrival in Cape Town, I moved in with my mom and stayed over at the prince's apartment while I looked for a place of my own. The prince said he didn't want us to be a live-in couple yet, and I accepted that because I didn't want to lose him. There wasn't the option of living again with my sister because she was traveling in India, and I didn't want to live in my mom's spare room. I went back to work at the hotspot bar and signed up to do a short photography course. I was relieved to be "home" again.

One week later, I decided that was the day that I would make the call. I was at my mom's apartment, and she had stepped out to buy groceries from the store. I paced up and down and practiced what I would say over and over. The piece of paper I held was wet from my sweaty fingers and creased from being scrunched up in my pocket. I sat down at my mom's rolltop desk near an open window. Palm trees rustled in the wind, and a ray of sunlight warmed my back. I dialed the number. A gentle, kind, calm voice answered. I told him my name. "I'm calling because I think I might have a problem," I said. He thanked me for calling him and told me it was okay to be nervous. He asked me how I got his number. I told him. "How about you come to our weekly support group? In fact, we are meeting tonight. Come. I'll see you there. Okay?" He sounded like he was in a hurry, and he gave me no time to think about it.

"Um . . . okay," I said.

He gave me the address and time of the meeting. I put the phone down and took a deep breath. I didn't know then that it was the most important call I would ever make. The sun reflected off the windowpane and shone light directly at me. I realized that for the first time in a decade, I had humbled myself enough to know that I needed help.

That night my mom drove me to a house opposite what I would discover later was a rehabilitation clinic. We parked in the brick driveway. She put her hand on mine and told me it would be okay. I sat with one hand on each knee, short of breath, my heart beating as fast as the train I heard going by in the distance. We watched a group of girls cross the road from the clinic. They huddled together like geese, clasping each other's arms. They wore cardigans and sweatshirts and baggy T-shirts and loose pants that sagged at the groin. Some had sunken cheeks, others frizzy hair, others bulging eyes. Some had a sad beauty, others a wrecked ugliness. Their hair was limp, their complexions pale, and their backs hunched. I watched as they followed each other through the door.

Every one of them was thin. My mom held my hand tight, but I pulled it away. She touched my face, and I could see she had tears in her eyes.

"I'll be here waiting for you when you come out," she said. "I love you."

I kicked open the car door and shut it hard behind me. I crossed my arms over my chest and marched to the front door and rang the doorbell. I looked back and saw my mother wiping her eyes. She smiled. Her lips quivered. She started up the engine, reversed the car, rolled down her window, waved, and blew me a kiss. *I love you*, she mouthed. The door opened. I walked inside. She drove off.

I entered a small room with windows along two walls and plastic chairs arranged in a circle. It was a room full of girls, some younger than me, some older. There was only one man. He had a thick head of brown hair, an angular face, and a masculine jawline. He smiled at me warmly as I walked in. He motioned to me to find a seat. I sat opposite the windows and waited for the shuffling to quiet down. Sitting there entangled in my body, uncomfortable in myself, an enormous wave of relief came over me, telling me it was going to be okay. I lifted both feet onto my chair and hugged them close to my body. I put my hands under my butt and sank into the chair. It was the first time, since the beginning of my anorexia, that I felt genuinely safe.

The man in the circle told everyone to quiet down and to sit properly with both feet on the ground and to stop fidgeting. It had been his voice that had welcomed me on the phone earlier in the day. I put my feet down and folded my bony arms over my concave belly. I wore a blue T-shirt with *Junior Sport* scribbled on it, the sleeves cut off at the shoulders and the bottom rim shredded. My baggy bell-bottom jeans hung well below my hipbones, which protruded like little rocks under my skin. My panties stuck out. My legs spiraled around one another like the roots of a twisted tree, and my feet were encased in black boots with soles thick enough to walk on hot coals.

The man introduced himself as Gregory. He was the clinic's psychologist and the support group's facilitator. I liked him immediately even though he did not bark orders and was gentle and kind. I was slowly letting down my guard and responding to softness. He smiled when he spoke and listened when others shared. He did not raise his voice or patronize or make any judgments. He went clockwise around the circle and asked each girl to introduce herself, to share a little bit about herself and to tell us why she was there.

When it came my turn to say my name aloud and speak my truth, my hands covered my eyes and tears poured out like heavy rain. I cried for the many years that I had denied myself the comfort of being supported and heard. The little girl in me sobbed with relief from the agony and desperation she had felt being starved all those years. I wept for the absolute futility—which I suddenly became aware of while sitting there among fellow sufferers—of having isolated myself and suffered alone. Deep in my heart I had known, all along, that reaching out for support might have ended it.

A few weeks later, my prince in leather pants set off on a spiritual sojourn in search of a shaman in the faraway hills, leaving his princess behind to set herself free.

Chapter Sixteen

ON THE ROAD

I wish I could say that everything changed after my first support group and that I immediately became a healthy new person. But it doesn't work that way. You don't give up something to which you are deeply committed, in which you have invested all your energies for so long, just like that. Yes, I wanted to be well. But I did not fully comprehend that it would mean letting anorexia go, as though she meant nothing.

After group that day, some of the girls stayed behind to talk to Gregory. He caught my eye as I stood up, motioned for me to walk toward him, and smiled. "Just a minute," he said. The girls finished talking to him and left. He lifted a leather-bound diary off the seat next to him and opened it up, and using his teeth he popped the lid off of his purple felt-tip pen.

"So let's arrange an appointment for you to see me as soon as possible. How does first thing Monday morning sound? Shall we make it at seven?"

I frowned.

"If that's too early, we can make it . . . let me see . . . I have a cancellation in the afternoon at three. Should we schedule you in then?"

"But I thought I was just coming tonight to this group," I told him.

"It's up to you. But I highly recommend that you consider seeing a psychologist for one-on-one weekly sessions. I am pretty booked up, but I do have these few slots available. Let me know, okay?"

He flapped his diary closed and smiled.

"Afternoon is better," I said, cracking my knuckles.

"All right, then." He lifted the long ribbon that opened his diary to the same page. "Three it is. I'll see you then." He gave me one last warm smile. "Please excuse me; I have to run. See you Monday."

Gregory disappeared down the stairs into the swarm of bumbling girls and left me standing there alone in my burst bubble. I didn't know then that this would be the man to hold my hand as I took my first steps out into the real world. It had not yet registered in my mind that I had started the recovery process. I was in no way prepared for what it would entail. I was just relieved to have found someone to whom I could vent my frustration on an intellectual level. And I hoped I would find the answer to why it started in the first place. A force greater than myself had taken over. And I went along with it, effortlessly, like a falling leaf. I had no idea where I was headed. But I knew something was coming. I just didn't know what. I left that day unaware that I was on the road; my journey had begun.

Gregory's therapy room was yellow—the color of emotions, according to the chakras. Two silky sofas with gold specks were neatly arranged around a glass coffee table with cream legs that made holes in the carpet. On the table rested a pad of paper set at a diagonal to the table edge, on top of which rested pink and purple felt-tip pens. My name was written in big round pink letters and was underlined in the top right-hand corner of the pad. In the center of the table was a white plastic Kleenex container with a thin slit on top. The paintings on the wall were spaced apart at perfect increments. Gregory's desk was tucked in the corner, and his chair was at a perpendicular angle to it. His lampshade was tilted at the exact right angle to allow just enough light, the window was ever so slightly ajar, and the air conditioner was on low, purring.

Gregory sat opposite me on the single-seat sofa and leaned forward to reach for the pad of paper on the coffee table. He set it down on a hardcover book on his lap.

"Let's get the technicalities out the way, shall we?" I reluctantly answered each of the following questions: "What is the correct spelling of your full name?" "Your date of birth, please?" "Tell me about your family." "Do any of them have a medical history I should know about?" "How old were you when your parents divorced?" "What does your mother do for a living?" "And your father?" "How many sisters and brothers do you have?" "How many years older or younger is she?" "What age were you when you moved to Israel and back? How old were you when you changed schools?"

He asked more questions, and, although I answered honestly, I couldn't help but think, *Boring. What the hell has this got to do with anything? I don't want to rehash the stupid chronology of my life and its geographical whereabouts and nuclear family crap! I want to get to the root of why I am here in the first place. I want ONE answer for the madness that is my life. And I want it NOW!*

For the rest of the session, Gregory continued to patiently ask me one question after another in an attempt to fill in the details of my life's history. I squirmed around in my seat, fidgeted with the throw cushions next to me and spat out each answer as quickly as I could just to get it over with as fast as possible so I could move on to what I believed was my motivation for being there.

Gregory noticed my frustration and said, "I am going to have to ask you to bear with me. I need to get a sense of your background before we can begin to move forward. This will not take too long. We will have all the time we need next week to start therapy."

"Next week? But I don't want to wait. I want to know why I am here now!"

"I understand," he said. "But you will have to wait. First things first, and then next week we can talk about everything else. We are going to have to wrap this session up now because I'm afraid our time is up."

I looked at his clock. The hand was one minute removed from the hour.

"We've still got one minute!" I snapped.

He smiled. "It will have to wait."

The next week I sat in his yellow room again, and nothing had changed except that there was no pad of paper on the table and no girly felt-tip pens.

"Aren't you going to write anything down?" I asked.

"Today we will just be talking," he explained.

There were a few seconds of silence, and then I said, "I have a confession to make. Last week when I was here, I didn't tell you that I had not slept at all the night before. I spent the whole night doing cocaine with my ex-boyfriend's friend. He lives in a mansion on the ocean. He offered me lines at the bar, and I couldn't say no. My boyfriend is out of town, and I miss him. I was lonely. So I went home with this guy. But I didn't sleep with him. We were coked up until sunrise."

I didn't know that it was the last time I would ever do cocaine.

"I see," he said. "Maybe we should start there." He straightened the collar of his shirt and pulled his V-neck cardigan further down over his stomach. "Would you like to tell me how cocaine makes you feel?"

I let my head drop to my shoulder, looked up, and thought about the question. "Carefree," I answered.

"What else?"

"It's fun. You know. It makes you spontaneous so you can let go."

"Don't you think you can be spontaneous and have fun and let go without it?"

"It's not the same."

I moved myself from the sofa seat to the floor and propped both arms on the glass coffee table and played with the Kleenex box.

"Do you always have fun on drugs?" he asked.

"No."

"Do you ever have fun off drugs?"

"No."

"Drugs obliterate your sense of being careful," he said. "Therefore, you may feel carefree, but you are actually being careless. To be carefree is to be spontaneous in your fun without being distracted by your responsibilities. It is suspending a heaviness."

Whatever. I still want to be carefree, whatever it means, I thought. "What if I'm just vain?" I asked.

"Well, what is vanity?" he countered.

"Vanity is egotistical. Arrogant. Selfish. Shallow. Superficial."

"Vanity is a protective sheath to cover up and protect you from resonating with the pain at a deeper level," he said. "Vanity denies access to the pain deep inside."

I don't want to analyze it; I just want you to tell me why all of this started in the first place. "Maybe I just like being thin," I snapped.

"Let's imagine a castle," he said, ignoring my statement. "The castle is surrounded by a moat, and in the moat is water. You built a big moat around your castle. But when the war is over, is the moat still necessary? Doesn't it become obsolete? Think of your anorexic body as the moat and the castle as your soul. You once were vulnerable and needed protection, from whatever the issues were, but do you still need that protection? And was it ever a protection in truth? Aren't you strong enough to grow up and face responsibility? Aren't you ready to become an adult? To be a woman?"

There was a long pause in the conversation after this. We had been talking for what seemed like ages as I had been writing everything down, word for word, knowing that I would want to read it over and over to try to make sense of what he was saying. For the rest of the session we sat in one long silent pause while I got up to open the window for fresh air, only to close it again a few seconds later, while I moved to sit from the sofa to the floor and then back on the sofa. I was so uncomfortable with the silence that I heard myself making trite small talk, mostly commenting on his anal nature and the quiet stillness in the room. "You are used to chaos," he said. Just then Gregory pointed to the clock on the wall to show me that it was time to wrap up our session.

"Have you called to make an appointment with the nutritionist I referred you to last week?"

"No. Not yet."

"It will be futile to pursue therapy if you do not see the nutritionist simultaneously."

"What's the point? I've been to one before. Besides, my food is fine."

"It's your choice," he said. "But I guarantee you that the one will not work without the other. Unfortunately, I cannot continue to see you anymore unless you make an appointment to work with her too. That is the rule."

I told Gregory that I would make an appointment with the nutritionist, and I said goodbye and left his office. That night, I wrote in my journal:

What if I let go of it? What part of me will die? Why can I not let go of it for anything? What part of me does this disorder define? Who will I be without it? What will I be? Where will I be? Responsibility. I will take control of my life.

On my first visit to the nutritionist, she told me to take off all my clothes except my bra and panties. She led me to a scale. She weighed me. *How absolutely absurd it is for me to weigh exactly the same as I weighed when I was fourteen—almost ten years ago*, I thought. *Because surely we grow; surely we grow up?* She thanked me, and I got dressed again. I wore a T-shirt that my mom bought me that was fit for a four-year-old, with a picture of Pooh Bear gauging a tub of honey, because she knew I envied his easygoing attitude. My mother never intended for me to wear it but I did and it set a trend of wearing children's shirts over the next couple of years. Maybe it was an unconscious attempt to stay childlike, but more than that I think the tightness felt comforting around my chest just as a baby feels calm and secure when swaddled tightly by a blanket. The nutritionist put her hand on my back and led me to my chair. I sat down and lifted my feet onto it and wrapped my arms around my shins.

Her room was decorated in bright colors—red, white, and blue—like a children's playroom. She sat opposite me, upright at her desk, and clasped her fingers as she leaned forward. Her thick natural blonde hair was pulled back in a neat ponytail. She wore a simple blouse and casual pants. She also didn't blink an eye when she saw my skin and bones. She was kind without being smothering; she didn't judge anything I said, and she had just the right amount of confidence to make me feel held without feeling intimidated. She made consistent eye contact and called me "sweetie" a lot.

This was a make-or-break meeting, and I trusted that she had my best interests in mind from the start. She knew why I was there even if I was oblivious to my own intention. Her role was to erode the stigma around my food issue and break it down into bits of manageable pieces for me to digest. After introducing herself as Tracey, she started to talk, and I tried to listen.

"You process your feelings through your weight." "Part of you is hiding behind the food." "When you start to eat, you will become full of feelings." "The food will ground you." "We have two nervous systems: the parasympathetic—which makes you feel grounded, full, calm, relaxed—and the sympathetic—which makes you feel high, empty, tense, jittery, starved." "Hunger will mean that your metabolism is working." "Delaying eating equals addiction." "You starve because you won't allow yourself to feel your feelings." "Your food is an expression of yourself."

I have absolutely no idea what this woman is talking about, I thought. *I've written it all down because I want to understand, and maybe one day it will make sense to me, but right now it doesn't. But she obviously knows what she's talking about. She's a nutritionist who sees girls like me every day. But what the fuck has my food got to do with my feelings? There is nothing wrong with my feelings. And there is nothing wrong with my food. It's under control. What does she mean that I starve because I won't allow myself to feel my feelings?*

Next, Tracey hooked me up to an elaborate device that

looked like a polygraph and stuck small patches all over my arms. Then she read some numbers off the machine.

"I am testing your body fat, body lean, body water, body mass, and metabolic rate, sweetie. That way I can estimate the average requirement of calories that you will need to eat in order to be at your lowest possible weight with the maximum nutrients."

She unhooked the spark plugs and sat behind her desk copying numbers from the machine onto a piece of paper.

"Just give me a second, sweetie, I'll be right with you . . ." She put her pen down and leaned forward with her fingers linked. A gold ring on her wedding finger glistened in the light.

"I am just letting you know . . ." she paused, then continued, "that you may put on between two and four pounds."

"No way!" I said, hugging my arms tighter around my body. "I can't put on weight. I'm not doing this. That's too much. I can't. I can't put on two to four pounds. I won't!"

Tracey sat still just looking at me. She expressed no pity or sympathy. She had a job to do, and if I was going to throw a temper tantrum like a toddler, then she would consider our meeting over. I stopped ranting and looked at her face. She seemed to care, but more like a teacher cares that you get good grades and pass the test than a mother who cares that you excel and fulfill your individualistic dreams. She had no more than half an hour and some tests invested in me. She knew it would be a waste of time to force, persuade, cajole, or bribe. What she was doing was leaving it all up to me. She gave me the responsibility to decide my fate and to face the consequences. She let me take control.

"It is entirely your choice," she said finally.

"Fine," I said softly, lowering my head and picking at the skin on my fingers. "But no more than four pounds!"

"Don't worry, sweetie, it will not be more. Okay?"

I looked up and nodded.

"Now, your homework for this week is to make a list of all the foods that you like to eat and to bring that list to me when I see you again in ten days."

What a lame request, I thought. *Why doesn't she just ask me to spit it out now? My list is short. It's always on the tip of my tongue. There is nothing that I am more certain of in the world than the content of my list. Surely she knows that. She must know it. It's not that I'm against making a list, it's just that it seems totally ridiculous to have to go home and think about it for more than one week when I can just list all the food that I eat on five fingers right here and right now!*

Exactly ten days later, I handed Tracey my list. She thanked me, set it down on her table, and started to write on another piece of paper, and then she glanced at my list and wrote some more. Once she was done, she lifted up her piece of paper as though it were a scroll or a certificate.

"There," she said. "This is your meal plan."

My meal plan? What the fuck is this? I'm not a psychotic patient in a lockdown unit that needs some stupid menu. I know what to eat every day.

"What for?" I asked.

"It is your suggested food intake for one day. In order to progress in recovery, you will need to follow a strict menu, and you will need to write down your food counts daily."

She handed me the paper, and one word at the top left side of the page jumped out at me: *PATIENT.* Next to it in pen was my name.

Oh my God! I can't believe it! This is me. This is my reality. This is what it has come down to. I am a patient. I am this patient. A sick patient. This is a doctor's room. This is my life. I scanned the paper from top to bottom, left to right, my eyes darting over the spiral flowers in the margins.

This is more food than I've eaten the whole week—or month, for that matter. I'm not kidding. Is this woman insane? There is so much food listed on this paper, and there are six times each day that I am supposed to eat it! Are you fucking mad? There is no way in hell that I am going to eat all this shit. It's just too much. Nobody in their right mind eats this much in one day. This is insane. Get me the fuck out of here. This is not normal.

"There is no way that I can eat this much," I said. "It is just not normal."

She looked me straight in the eye and did not flinch. "Sweetie, you can eat it, and you will. You'll see."

Our time was up.

Tracey walked me out of her office, with her arm around my shoulder, and told her secretary to book me another slot for the following week. I took one step out into the piercing daylight and burst into tears. Couldn't she see that by eating her meal plan I'd be admitting defeat? And that would make the past decade futile. I clutched my meal plan written on beige paper, with its flowers spiraling around the edges, neatly fitted into its blue transparent mental-patient envelope. I stood on the sidewalk in the heat, my head spinning. Tears gushed like a burst pipe. What would I turn to now?

The following table was my suggested meal plan for one day. My food choices were broken up into four groups: carbohydrates (CHO), protein (PRT), fat (FAT), and fruit (FRU). Every day, my challenge was to eat the right amount of units—that Tracey had calculated was needed for my body's caloric intake—for my three meals, three snacks, and an after-dinner treat. (1 CHO or 1 PRT or 1 FAT or 1 FRU was equal to one unit.)

Note: 30g portion of food = size of a matchbox

Breakfast – 08h00:
4 CHO + 2 FAT eg. 1 cup muesli
1 PRT eg. 1 cup 2% milk

Snack – 11h00:
3 FRU eg. 1.5 cups fruit juice

Lunch – 13h00:
3 CHO eg. 1 ciabatta roll
2 PRT + 2 FAT eg. 60g cheddar cheese + free salad
2 FAT eg. 2 teaspoons butter

Snack – 15h00:
1 PRT + 2 FAT eg. 30g peanuts
2 FRU eg. 2 apples

Dinner – 19h00:
3 PRT eg. 90g fish
3 CHO eg. 1 cup cooked rice + free veggies/salad
1 FRU eg. 1 banana

After dinner:
3 CHO eg. 3 shots tequila

Late-night snack:
3 CHO eg. 1 ciabatta roll
1/2 PRT + 1/2 CHO eg. 2 tablespoons hummus

In order for my body to function normally again, I needed to eat a certain number of units from each food group to meet my daily total. There was also the miscellaneous list, which allowed me to drink alcohol. Three shots of tequila featured on my meal plan as an after-dinner snack because Tracey said I would drink it anyway. But it was the combination foods list, which mixed and matched fats and carbohydrates, that scared me most. On my third visit, I argued against it.

"Why do I need to eat the combination foods?" I said. "It's not like ice cream is healthy. None of the food on that list is healthy. Why should I pump my body full of empty calories when I could feed it more nutritionally? What's the point of stuffing myself with chips and cakes and cookies and puddings? Ice cream is just not healthy! I mean, what's the point?"

"There is no point," Tracey answered. "But isn't it only normal to be lying on the beach with some friends on a hot day eating a popsicle, or to drop into the store to buy an ice cream cone when you are walking around town? That is what normal people do, and there is no reason why you shouldn't be doing that too."

A couple of weeks later, Tracey showed me my chart. She had worked out the calculations according to the reading on my "polygraph" test at my first appointment. She then used my height and weight to determine my body mass index (BMI). Here's what my chart said:

FAT
PATIENT'S VALUES: KG 5.6 (12.3 pounds): 10.6%
NORMAL VALUES: 20–26%

LEAN
PATIENT'S VALUES: KG 47.4 (104.5 pounds): 89.4%
NORMAL VALUES: 74–80%

TOTAL BODY WATER
PATIENT'S VALUES: KG 33.51 (73.9 pounds): 63.2%
NORMAL VALUES: 50–60%

BASAL METABOLIC RATE
KJ: 6561
KCals: 1568

ESTIMATED AVERAGE REQUIREMENT
KJ: 10498
KCals: 2509

BODY MASS INDEX
PATIENT: 18.1
NORMAL: 18–25

It was only years into recovery that I realized the significance of calculating an anorexic's body mass index. A BMI lower than 18 would classify you as medically malnourished and make you eligible for admission to a rehabilitation clinic. A BMI of 18 or higher would make you qualified to cohabit with citizens of the normal world. At the time that I started recovery, my BMI was 18.1, so I was borderline. Had I begun recovery a few months earlier—or even weeks earlier—I may have been admitted as an inpatient to the rehabilitation clinic. Instead, I was sent out into the real world to confront my feelings and stand on my own two feet—even if I was barefoot in a new world made of broken glass.

Chapter Seventeen

SKY IS FALLING

In the first couple of months of recovery, it felt as though all I did was eat. Breakfast, snack, lunch, snack, dinner, snack, snack. My entire life seemed to revolve around the meal plan. Eating took up so much time and energy.

I had moved into a semi-detached home in the Muslim quarter of the city, high on a hillside, and I found a housemate to share the rent. My bedroom was painted a happy yellow. The sun-kissed kitchen had retro vinyl floors and opened out onto a small, square yard with walls painted cloudy blue as though the sky had fallen and splashed all over them. My housemate and I hung colorful Mexican hammocks above the potted plants in the yard, in which we spent many days doing tarot-card readings and gossiping about our unrequited love with our princes. Every night, I worked at the bar, and the rest of the time I spent alone at home with my meal plan.

My mission every single day was to ensure that I consumed my allocated units of carbs, proteins, fats, and fruits—not a unit more or a unit less—the sum of which made up my food counts for the day. This way, I would not put on weight too quickly, nor would I lose weight. Every night, I prepared my menu for the following day. I chose my food and its portions according to the units on the meal plan. And the following day, I ate exactly what I had planned to eat the night before in order to make up my counts, and I wrote it all down throughout the course of the day. There was one rule: to consume my total food counts, which remained the same, every single day. And to stay within that boundary. No matter what.

The meal plan was a perfect regimen for a recovering anorexic like myself who thrived on meticulous calculations and doted on perfectionism. It gave structure to my day. It contained me. As long as I was counting and calculating, I felt I was getting somewhere. I had purpose. It was similar to the attempts I had made in my own mind over the years, only this time I was consuming rather than abstaining. Even though I hated the act of eating—the tastes were unfamiliar, and there was no pleasure in it—I persisted because I had made up my mind: I wanted to be well. Food was simply fuel to keep me going so I could get to the other side. Escape my past. Start over.

At the bar, I worked nights with another bartender about my age. She was a sexy young woman with short, slick black hair and a hot figure, who clearly had no such issues with food. I envied her. How at the start of every shift, she strolled into the bar, carrying a meal she had just purchased on her way. I remember one night in particular when she brought in what looked to me like a giant sandwich. She unwrapped it, took a huge bite, smacked her lips, and set it down again. In between wiping down the bar counter, stacking the clean glasses and chatting, she would casually grab her sandwich, take more huge bites, smack her lips again, and continue alternating bites with her duties until she had consumed the entire thing. She made eating look so easy, and so enjoyable.

Meanwhile, I spent my days walking in and out of the

kitchen to get food, prepare food, and eat food. And nothing else. Three times a day plus snacks. And in the spaces between, I sat on the vinyl floor in the sun, hunched over my blue file totaling my counts, calculating my sanity. I was a mental patient walking from the inside to the outside, to the inside to the outside, with her blue folder tucked under her arm. Her security blanket. All I needed was a mauve terry cloth bathrobe and an IV drip and bad TV, and I would have been set to act out the clichéd role of insanity.

I ate methodically. I took two slices of whole wheat seed bread out the package. I spread a carefully measured teaspoon of butter. I sliced a particular amount of cheese, chopped some herbs and a tomato, and broke off some pieces of lettuce. I walked outside into the backyard and sat cross-legged on the concrete ground and set my plate down in front of me. I took a few deep breaths, banged my chest with my palm to quell the rising panic, took a tiny bite, and swallowed. I felt as though I were losing myself with each bite. The person I had become—anorexia.

As food worked its way into my psyche and my body, my numb, petrified emotions sought refuge deep within. Then slowly, slowly, parts of me began to dissolve, and pain filtered in like drip coffee. I was told to sit with the pain, the deep, infected pain that I had stored for years. Pain that was confusing. Pain that was elusive. I was told just to sit with it as though it were a sick pet.

There were no bandages, ointments, stitches, or morphine to ease the pain. Had I undergone surgery for broken bones, I would have been told to lie in bed, recover, doctor's orders, and people would have sashayed in to visit and sit by my bedside and spoil me with gifts and hold my hand and wipe my brow. But there I was, suddenly sober in the real world without my fix, without my starvation. And I must have looked pretty ordinary. Like there was nothing wrong with me except that I was a bit on the thin side. But I was lost. I had been abandoned in the wrong reality. And nobody could see that I didn't belong. Had I broken my bones, I would have been in bed recovering. But I had broken my soul, fractured my personality, and torn apart my identity. It would take a lot longer than a few months of bed rest to heal.

"All I do is eat!" I told Gregory at one of our weekly sessions.

I sat on the edge of the sofa, slumped into the cushion with my elbows on my knees and my chin buried in my hands.

"It only feels that way because your life has been so consumed by your obsession with food for so long. This is just your body's way of adjusting," he said. "It will soon pass, and there will invariably be time and space for life."

Gregory wore his usual bottle-green cardigan and brown leather shoes. His laces were done up in perfect bows, and his socks matched the design on the sofa.

"I have to tell you, I fucked up the last two days," I blurted out. "I didn't follow my meal plan. It was my twenty-fourth birthday. There was pressure. I didn't eat breakfast. I didn't eat lunch. At four in the afternoon, I was so famished I scarfed down whatever was in the fridge, and then I felt fat and full and heavy and burdened and emotional and chaotic. Now I feel like such a failure."

"It is important for you to remember that if your meal plan has lapsed for a day or two, you don't have to cram all the missed meals into one evening. Instead, just let it go and pick it up again according to your meal plan the next day," he said.

I nodded, sat up, and slouched against the sofa armrest. "It was skipping breakfast that set me off track. And then I was so upset and angry with myself, and then I just can't eat when I'm crying."

"Breakfast does set the tone for the day. It is an important meal," he said. "Just don't beat yourself up about it, and forge ahead as you were doing."

His voice was calming and reassuring, and I wished he would scoop me up in his arms and hug me.

"I'm struggling to eat this week—I'm using a lot. I'm scared this is how it will be for the rest of my life. That I will never be able to manage anything other than eating three meals a day. I will never have a boyfriend, a family, a job, a hobby—all because I am too busy eating!"

I threw my arms up in the air and collapsed back on the sofa. "Look at me! I'm too bloody exhausted to sit up. This is sucking all my energy!"

"Think of it this way," he said, flashing his sweet smile. "You have two selves inside—the destructive and the constructive. Right now, you are fighting inside to let go of the one and to welcome the other."

"But why must it be such a struggle?" I said.

"Because you are afraid to let go. The reason has to do with your fear of entering into unknown territory—your healthy, normal, well, stable side. All your life you have been familiar with unstable things. This spice, decadence, addiction that you seek has become familiar and exciting, but there are healthy things that can bring you true happiness, which you are afraid to embrace because it is unfamiliar."

"Like what?" I asked. I sat forward to catch the true meaning of the word *happiness* for the first time.

"Like safety, and security, and stability," he said.

I sat back, quiet, still. "Oh. I never thought of that."

"We all have different perceptions of words depending on

what headspace we are in and how we have been shaped by our backgrounds, our upbringing, what we have been exposed to." He went on and then finished his thought. I sat for a minute in silence contemplating. Then I said, "I've got one for you. What's your idea of decadence?"

I anticipated something in line with my version: slinky lines of cocaine on a marble slate and tequila shots slammed until the bottle is sapped of its last golden drop.

"A bubble bath," he said.

My jaw dropped wide open. I was speechless. I just burst out laughing and laughed and laughed while Gregory sat still watching me, amused.

"It looks like you find my answer amusing?" he said, without any defensiveness in his voice. We both smiled. This was a huge session in that we were really talking about deep, entrenched issues that I had never addressed with anyone, let alone acknowledged myself. One of the things I valued most about Gregory was his ability to have intellectual conversations that stimulated my mind. Slowly, slowly he was ever so lightly cracking my hard shell and I didn't even know it. He managed to cut through all my defenses and pretenses and challenge me at a time when I desperately needed to take a look inside myself. I am so grateful that I wrote down verbatim so much of our conversations in those sessions because he was so right in his assessments. His gentle way and his astute insights guided me along on my journey back to myself. Gregory saved my life.

I had my routine set in the first three months of recovery: psychologist once a week, support group once a week, dietician once every ten days, bar shifts six times a week, exercise every other day, three meals a day and snacks in between. My housemate was instrumental in helping me prepare my meals. We made it a ritual. Often we shopped together for food. Supermarkets were a barrage of products, smells, deep freeze, bakery, raw meat, and labels upon labels that I had once known by heart, words and numbers that had dictated my life, abolished my feelings. My housemate took the pressure off me and made decisions regarding what to purchase. Restaurants were still enemy territory. It felt safer to eat at home, to prepare the food myself, to know how it would look, how big a portion would be, and how it would taste. Eating out posed too many choices. I didn't know yet what I liked, and I couldn't tolerate too much tastiness.

"But food is pleasurable," Gregory once said. "It is not just a prophylactic to stuff down your throat so that you don't relapse."

Although I only put on between two and four pounds in the first few months, just like Tracey had promised, my attitude toward my body image changed overnight. Food suddenly grounded me in a more humble and less flaunted reality. The shift happened one night when I was working late at the bar. The place was packed with sex and seduction, beer and corruption, and I worked the bar wearing tight tie-dye bell-bottoms and a tiny top with a knot tied in front to show off my stomach. A woman sauntered up to the bar. She had roasted skin, a low-cut mini skirt that nearly revealed her pubic hairline, a belly chain that dangled down her crotch, and a boob tube that squeezed her breasts into prominent cleavage that looked like a raging river ran through it. She leaned over the bar, and behind her the boozers' jaws dropped when they caught a glimpse of her G-string sticking up her crack. The men shoved one another to move a step closer to her sickly sweet perfume and her horsetail hair. Their eyes burrowed deep down her cleavage and settled at her nipples. I felt disgusted by what I saw. I didn't want to be like this woman. A piece of meat. Objectified by men who meant nothing to her and cared less. I put my hands over my stomach and untied the knot in my shirt. It was my first sober taste of shame.

"Something shifted last night," I told my housemate the next morning over our ritual cup of instant coffee and a cigarette. "The slut in me is gone."

"Really? Well maybe I can get all her old clothes," she said.

"I mean it. I can't dress like that anymore, like a slut. It's gone: that sexuality, that lust, that spunk . . . gone. I'm twenty-fucking-four! I'm not a teenybopper anymore, and I don't want to be the archetypal whore."

My housemate grabbed my hand and dragged me to my overflowing wardrobe of juvenile apparel. She suggested that we sift through every single item of clothing and create a slut pile to give away and a humble pile to keep. Later she knocked on my door to give me a purple gemstone that she had picked up on a trip in India. I found out that it was an amethyst stone like those used in ancient Rome to ward off intoxication. The name is derived from the Greek word *amethustos*, which means not drunken or inebriated. It is also known as the "Sobriety Stone." It must have worked because soon after she gave it to me, I stopped drinking, but the more I sobered up, the worse I felt emotionally.

Today was bad, but tomorrow is a new day. Every day I wish to get through this because I cannot do it on my own. I wish to get through it so I can be free and whole. What is whole? I am exhausted —physically and emotionally and mentally exhausted. Please help me to end this struggle, help me to eat in moderation. I feel lost and directionless, like nine years ago in my existential phase. Everything is black and bleak. I don't want to feel this way; I only want to be happy. But I guess I'm trying to heal. These are such early days. I just wish this pain would go away. I've been undergoing an operation for ten years, an operation on my fucking soul, and these doctors just send me home with my blue file as though I'll be better tomorrow. This is my fucking life! Where is everybody? Does everybody feel this way? What is this pain? What the fuck is hurting so bad? Never before have I felt so desperate for help from up above. This fear, uncertainty, not knowing is eating me alive. Where is the security, the structure, the containment of anorexia? I am filled with fear of the world. I am so scared to feel this way. So scared this feeling will never ever go away.

One sunny afternoon, my housemate was out. It was lunchtime, and I had prepared a sandwich and had stepped outside to eat it in the backyard in front of the fallen sky on the walls. I sat on the ground and laid the plate next to me. I banged my chest and took a deep breath, picked up the sandwich, took a bite, and fell forward like someone had hit me on the back with a wooden plank and knocked me over. I was facedown sobbing, cupping my eyes with my hands, and rocking to and fro. Tears gushed. A sharp pain stabbed me in the chest. It was a deeply embedded pain, like my heart was being ripped apart, like my soul was thrashing. My cries reverberated like the Islamic call to prayer in the nearby mosque. I started to pray out loud for the first time. I prayed in Hebrew. I prayed to Jesus. Krishna. Buddha. Allah. HaShem. The Divine Spirit. I prayed. And I sobbed.

Nobody warned me that when I gave up anorexia, I would die. I was angry with Gregory for not preparing me. For not sitting me down and saying, "Listen, I have something to tell you. You know this person that you have worked so hard to become, this person that you gave up your life for, that you sacrificed your soul for? She is going to die, and it will hurt more than you will be able to bear. You will wake up one morning and not know who you are. You will wake up and realize that without your anorexic persona, you have no identity, and you will feel lost and desperate, and your despair will become intolerable, and you will want to die again and again, but you will already be dead because anorexia was all you knew. You will need to know this and be prepared for your own death, and be prepared to live through it."

He never told me that. And how could he have? How can anyone prepare you to remain alive through your own death? I just wish he would have said, "You will start to feel things for the first time—feelings that you have been avoiding for the last ten years—and you will want to run away. You will want to hide, you will want to drink, you will want to do anything not to feel. So be careful who you invite into your life during this time. Be careful what you choose to believe. Be careful how you choose to find meaning in this confusion. Be careful what comes your way to offer you the identity, the truth, the meaning you will be desperately searching for."

But even if he had explained this word for word, I wouldn't have understood it. All I knew was that I had suddenly lost my identity, and I wanted out. I wanted salvation from the pain. But I knew that starving would just take me back to square one, and I was desperate enough to be committed to wanting a new beginning. So I clung to whatever I could to offer me an alternative to the pain. I clung to bar work. And above all, I clung to the manager at work who controlled the bar. I clung to him like my new life depended on it, which it did.

He was a positive influence in terms of my food and my sobriety because he ate three healthy meals a day and didn't touch alcohol. It was soon after we hooked up that I decided to stop drinking. It felt like a natural extension of my letting go of what I was starting to see as my debauched side. He took me to the same small deli for lunch and dinner every day and sat with me patiently while I scribbled down my food counts. It was the first time in years that I went willingly out to eat and actually ate substantial meals. What helped was that it was a tiny, family-owned Greek deli with a beautiful view of the mountain and only a handful of quaint tables outside on the sidewalk. The entire menu consisted of about eight dishes that were displayed in the deli counter. Every day there were the exact same dishes that you could clearly see through the glass counter. This helped eliminate unwanted surprises, as I knew each time what to expect from the food. I alternated between the tuna casserole and the vegetarian lasagna with a side salad and the consistency offered me a sense of safety I was desperately seeking in my new relationship with food. That deli was a godsend.

Yet despite all the positives, again I found myself immersed in a guy's life and forgot that I was supposed to be living my own. He was an exercise and health fanatic who trained every day lifting weights, boxing, or running laps around a field. I took up kickboxing and jogged with him and punched some bags. We had picnics in sunny parks like an elderly couple. We slept in the mornings, exercised in the afternoons, went to work at 5:00 p.m., and got home at 5:00 a.m. He carried knives and a gun on his person, which made me feel safe and secure. Protected. But the main reason I clung to him was because he offered me the opportunity to open my heart—to Jesus Christ. He was a devout reborn Christian who offered me an identity when I needed it most.

I was the reborn's bible baby. He bought me my own New Testament, with all of Jesus's words italicized in red. When I wasn't working on my meal plan, I sat in my backyard for hours on end reading Jesus's wisdom, trying to relate his words to my own agony, hoping to find hope beyond blind faith. On Sundays I accompanied the reborn to his church service, which was my substitute for raves—the Holy Spirit was my new ecstasy; the hymns were my new house music. People smiled, stretched out their arms, and were welcoming, praising, adoring, accepting. I felt safe. One morning, as I stood in the auditorium, tears streamed down my face as I sang the chorus of a hymn: "I can't walk this road alone . . ."

I needed to believe in something because I couldn't find the strength to believe in me, to have hope in something because I couldn't trust myself. I wanted to know that I would survive. Most of all, I wanted answers to my pain. This desire alone drove my recovery. *If I can just understand it*, I thought, *then I can let it go*. And so I decided, after much deliberation and countless conversations with the reborn, that I would ask Jesus into my heart and that I would do it properly, in a church, in front of witnesses. It would help me find the answers. It would save me from my pain.

"Jesus loves you!" "Amen." "Jesus loves you!" "Amen." "I said praise the Lord—Jesus loves you!" "AMEN." A skinny preacher stood on the stage in a hall with over two hundred chairs arranged in a semicircle surrounding the podium. I squeezed through the packed aisles of praising fans that threw their arms up in worship, their palms turned toward the stage like hundreds of stop signs. Looming above the preacher were high-tech flat-screen TVs that showed a video of churchgoers donating shoes to underprivileged children. Every "Praise the lord—Jesus loves you" from the manic preacher in the spotlight was echoed with "Amen" by the excited crowd.

"I call out to every one of you to ask the Lord into your hearts today so that you may be happy, you may be rich, you may get that raise. Now I'm going to ask you to step up to the front of the stage. That's right, if you feel it in your hearts, you just come on up to the front of the stage. That's right, people. And I am sure that not one of you here with us tonight knew that you would be standing up here tonight. This, my friends, is the power of the Holy Spirit. This is the power of the Lord, to help us to open our hearts. Amen. Because Jesus died to save us from our sins. Amen."

I stepped up to the front of the stage, as I had planned to do nights before, and felt a tepid heat rising from the small crowd of people gathered round me and the other twenty people in front of the stage. Their arms were outstretched, and their palms faced my back; their eyes were shut, and they were concentrating intently. The crowd closed in on us, holding their hands inches away from our bodies. Standing there as a Jew in my trance sweatshirt with tribal patterns snaking up my arms and my wild hair, I felt wrong. Like I was imposing, trespassing.

"Brace yourselves, my friends, for you are about to receive the Lord Jesus Christ into your hearts tonight."

We were shuffled away from the stage through a small door at the back of the amphitheater. It was a square room, with brick walls and no windows, devoid of ventilation. A blackboard flanked one wall, and gray plastic chairs were arranged in a row before it. We took our seats. Men in suits charged in and stood before us in a row. Equal spacing separated their patent leather shoes. Their hands were clenched in fists in front of their groins. They were gray men, with gray hair, gray skin, gray suits, gray energy, and white nametags pinned to their pockets. We were then cordoned off into smaller groups, females separated from males. I joined three women, including a woman wearing a nametag whose job it was to explain to us what had just happened. Speaking with a strong Portuguese accent, she told us to refer to our Bibles and to hold hands and pray.

"Only Jesus can save you," she said.

But I interrupted and asked, "Why?"

"Because, only Jesus can save you—it is written here in the Bible."

"But don't you think we can save ourselves?"

"No," she said, pointing to the line that she repeated over and over and pressing her finger deeper onto the page. "We are here to be saved by our Lord Jesus Christ."

"Saved from what?" I asked.

Her answer was the same: "Saved from our sins because only Jesus can save you—it is written here in the Bible."

She tapped the line on the page like she was punching stubborn keys on a keyboard. She told us to hold hands again and commence the prayer, but I broke the link when she said to repeat after her, "I belong to Jesus." Then we were shuffled back out the small door into a supposedly new world. On our way out, she stood at the door and gave each of us a handout to take home. When it was my turn to leave the room, she looked away and handed me a booklet. I tucked it under my arm and exited the door smiling. On the bright red cover were the words *CHOOSE LIFE*.

Chapter Eighteen

I don't know whether Jesus entered my heart in that church, but after that day, I started to experience little serendipitous happenings. Call it luck, fate, or synchronicity. Maybe a higher power was taking care of me because I was starting to take care of myself.

Throughout the following year I would vacillate between embracing positive, healthy, inspiring things and negative, decadent, abusive things. Both sides would be alluring, but in the end, in a strange twist of fate, the one to prevail over the other would lead me to real recovery.

Just before my churchgoing letdown, about three months after my first therapy session, my father had called. I had probably spoken to him on and off on the phone and maybe seen him a few times since I moved to Cape Town. I don't remember much more than that. He told me he was leaving for New York City in a few days' time to go on a weeklong business trip and asked me if I wanted to go with him. I accepted his invitation, and then I put down the phone and sobbed. It would be an opportunity to bond with my father ten years after my anorexia started. Going to New York City again would be like coming full circle, since the time he took me there when I was fourteen. My sister would meet us there after her travels in India. The trip would be a welcome respite from the pain of recovery.

I said goodbye to the reborn, told the bar I was taking a week off work and got another bartender to cover for me, and soon enough I was in New York City, high on the reality of skyscrapers and consumer madness. I was hooked on the rush, the pace, the wild sea of faces. I used New York like a substance. I felt alive after leaving my emotions behind on Gregory's couch, even though he had cautioned me about going because he said it could pose a risk of a relapse. My father and I bonded just as I had hoped. I had always preferred him when he was on vacation. It was the only time he was present with me and undistracted by his businesses. Plus, the fact that I was now in recovery meant that I was starting to relate differently too. Being with him in New York for that week was exactly what I had needed to begin to feel some connection without the loaded resentment.

"I'm staying on," my sister said before our week was up. "Come on, let's fulfill our longtime dream of living together in a New York loft!"

I emailed Gregory to ask his opinion. *I would not recommend that you stay longer*, he wrote. *It may prove to be detrimental to your recovery. There is a strong chance that you could relapse because of the lack of support and familiarity.*

He was right. I knew that by running away, I was delaying and endangering the recovery process. But I would also be taking things a step at a time, knowing that some day I would have to go home to confront why it all started in the first place.

Three months of therapy is not enough to deal with any real emotions because when you surface from—in your case—a decade-long eating disorder, in order not to flood yourself with feelings, you go numb, he wrote. *But only after that do you start the real work.*

I knew there was no way I could just put all those years behind me and move on. I could not all of a sudden be a functioning adult, take full responsibility for myself, be creative, and have healthy relationships and love myself. But even one week away felt a lot better than the flood of agony that made me buckle over and pray in my backyard. So I decided to stay.

My father returned to South Africa, and my sister rented us a loft apartment in SoHo. Our flatmate gave me a complimentary membership to a hotspot yoga studio. My sister also found me a job waiting tables at a family-owned Italian restaurant in Chelsea whose motto was: "No Diet Coke—No decaf—No skim milk—Only good food." At the restaurant I ate everything on the menu from orechiette with broccoli rabe and sausage to penne vodka with pancetta to fried chicken Milanese to carpaccio and arugula salad. Nobody knew I was a recovering anorexic with a meal plan. They just saw me as a twenty-something foreigner with a healthy appetite and a lust for rich, tasty food, which I was starting to really enjoy. The chef felt like a father figure to me and I looked forward to him cooking me a special meal every time I worked. It felt like he was taking care of me, which was what I needed. I indulged in countless self-help books on healing with names like *Earth Medicine*, *Where Two Worlds Touch*, and *Sacred Mirrors*. I became deeply infatuated with the six-foot-tall Italian manager, whose mere existence was my inspiration to go to work every day. And one morning out of the blue I stopped smoking cigarettes and never looked back.

I was suddenly reinvented. I pretended that I was normal—pretended that I was a new person with no pain, with no past. A person who had never known anorexia. When I eventually told the restaurant's owner that I was an anorexic in recovery, she choked. She said that judging from the way I ate, she doubted it.

As I mentioned, because the chef prepared whatever I wanted to eat from the menu and his cooking was consistent in quality and taste, it made me feel safe in my new relationship with food. The predictability of the meals he prepared, and the fact that it was a substitute for me having to shop and cook for myself, eliminated a lot of stress, that in retrospect I know I wouldn't have been able to handle. After six months in New York, I stopped writing down my food counts. I felt I had enough practice with my meal plan to know what my body felt like eating rather than what it was prescribed. I ate happily, even though I put on a few more pounds. Food was becoming part of life.

One afternoon my sister surprised me with a three-day vacation in Mexico, where we would spend our time in the desert searching for the hallucinogenic cactus peyote. The cactus is renowned for invoking a deep spiritual connection with one's self and an abandonment of the ego. It is said to clear the mind and open it up to a higher consciousness. On our arrival, we found a local man at a store and asked him to drop us off in his pickup truck in the middle of the desert where he pointed out the Peyote cactus growing in the ground. After he left, we chopped it up with a pocket knife and tried to eat it along with orange slices and pieces of chocolate to hide its bitter taste. On our first night alone in the desert, while tripping on Peyote, I asked my sister to cut off all my hair, and we burnt it in the fire that we made. It was a symbolic gesture of me letting go of my old self and embracing a new self, even if it was, what felt to me like, a less-attractive one. It was another step toward a deeper appreciation of myself as a human being, as a spirit within a body.

On our return to New York, however, I found myself home alone one night. I looked at myself in a full-length mirror and I did not like what I saw. I ran my hands through the sticky gel in my cropped hair and grabbed at my new clothes that felt too tight all over my new weight. I picked at the pimples that sprouted on my once-flawless complexion. My sister walked in, and I collapsed onto the bed.

"I hate putting on this weight. I hate my hair. I hate what I look like," I cried. "I feel bloated and ugly and uncomfortable. I feel fat!"

She put her arms around me and held me tight. "It's only for now. Things will change. It's just an adjustment. You don't look ugly or fat, you just look different. Give it time," she said.

She reached into her bag and took out a pale pink envelope with dried flowers embedded in the paper.

"Happy nine-month anniversary of recovery," she said, hugging me tighter.

I wanted to cry, but I had no tears. "Nobody will love me if I look like this," I said.

"You're right," she said.

"First you have to learn to love yourself no matter what you look like."

She got up to make us a stir-fry for dinner and took an ice-cold beer out of the refrigerator.

"Here's to your recovery," she said, holding up her bottle in the air. "Cry, complain, shop—do what you have to—but things will change, and you will feel different. You'll see. That's the nature of transformation."

My sister had left India with a shaven head and a talisman around her neck and was now cocktail waitressing at a New York nightclub with an eyebrow ring and spiky dyed-black hair. *If anybody knows about change*, I thought, *she does*. She left me alone in the room and walked off to the kitchen. I opened the envelope she had given me and took out the letter she had written to me. It said that everyone, including herself, was so proud of me and rooting for me to get well. I wanted to believe the words, to feel them, but I felt numb and detached. I set the letter aside and picked up the journal next to my bed. I drew a line down the middle of the page, and in the top left corner I wrote *Old body*, and underneath it I drew an outline of my thin anorexic body with no shape, just long lines and long hair down to the pinched waist. In the top right corner I wrote *New body*, and underneath I drew an outline of a shapely, fuller body and short, stubbly hair. I compared the two images and decided that although I hated my new body, I did not want to go back to the way I was. So much good was happening on the inside that I went with it and trusted the universe to guide me through.

One of the most important catalysts to my transformation was yoga. I started the practice a few years earlier during the peak of my anorexia. My sugar daddy's sister had recommended that I try her yoga class and I have no idea what compelled me to go at the time. I had sauntered into class ready to mock the tradition and laughed when the yogis chanted *Om*. But when I stretched into various asana poses like downward dog, head stand, shoulder stand, and lotus pose, I often had to run to the restroom to cry from the physical pain of opening my heart and starting to let go. The pain continued for years, and ironically, it was that pain that kept me dedicated to the practice. Years later, after stopping and starting yoga again and again, I began to feel a subtle shift happening. I stopped commanding my body to do what I wanted it to do and learned to accept its limitations and above all to listen to what my body needed to do. Although aerobics, drugs, and raving loosened me up and allowed me to let go, they did so by inducing altered states of consciousness, whereas yoga created a centered state of awareness—of my self, my body, and my breathing.

Throughout my anorexia my rounded shoulders protected my heart, my caved-in chest prevented deep breathing, and my whole body locked up to stop me feeling the pain of my emotions. Yoga had the opposite effect. I slowly learned that I did not need to force or push my body to perform. By breathing into each pose, my body learned to let go at its own pace. I started to become aware of how my body felt and moved as opposed to being obsessed with how it looked and operated. It was a gradual process of unblocking and letting go that allowed my body to relax enough for me to start connecting with my inner self. Each breath calmed me down, centered me, and stopped the negative mind talk. During my practice, my mind was elsewhere. It was not concentrated on spiraling thoughts of consumption and feelings of guilt. Yoga helped me to confront myself rather than escape what I felt inside. Eventually, I realized that if I could apply the same dedication, discipline, and commitment to my yoga practice as I did to my starving regime, then it could steer me away from my destructive patterns.

A holistic yoga practice involves focusing awareness on the release of different energy centers—or *chakras*, as they are known in Sanskrit—of which there are seven located throughout the body. I learned that the fifth Chakra (*Vishuddha*), located at the throat, governs one's willpower, choosing between right and wrong, communication, creativity, and self-expression. The third Chakra (*Manipura*), located in the solar plexus, relates to one's sense of self, personal power, self-esteem, responsibility, and being easily upset by criticism. I was amazed to realize that anorexics' lives are focused entirely on restricting these two energy centers. Anorexics deprive themselves of food, which in turn causes a sensation of the throat closing, which in turns prevents food from making its way into the stomach and nourishing the whole body. On an energetic level, this translates to anorexics essentially using their indomitable willpower to block their communication, prevent creativity, and deprive themselves of their personal power and self-esteem, thus harming and limiting their sense of self.

So, while living in New York, I went to yoga classes every other day. As my mind started to calm down, I could absorb concepts and ideas a lot more. After class, I went to browse the esoteric section of the nearby bookstore that sold Buddha statues, *I Ching* coins, Indian incense and, tongue scrapers, among other things. I bought one book after another on women's health and emotional healing and creative visualization. I did inner-child exercises and made lists of adjectives describing myself in a positive light and drew pictures of how I perceived my old and new self from head to toe. I visualized pink bubbles filled with my intentions and meditated on bright light and my pain disappearing. I did invocations calling forth the powers to help me usurp their divine qualities and attempted clearings, where I tried to get in touch with blockages that were holding me back. I did tarot readings and picked the card of sexuality, among others, reminding me to heal sexual wounds from the past. I did loving affirmations telling myself over and over again that I deserve love and I deserve sexual pleasure. And I made myself a personal creed: to think positively, to be aware in every moment, to trust the perfection, and to nourish my self. I made it my soul mission to understand where I was. And only later, on my return to therapy, would I begin to focus on how I got there and why.

One night I did a reading from the *I Ching*—an ancient Chinese book, the oldest of the Chinese classics, called *The Classic of Changes*—that my sister bought me as a recovery gift. It came wrapped up in a parcel with double-sided copper coins that had Chinese engravings. My sister had written instructions on how to throw the coins and predict my luck. It was similar to doing a tarot reading and was determined by how the coins landed, which resulted in you having to read the text of one symbol. There were sixty-four symbols, each one a square shape consisting of different combinations of six stacked horizontal black lines. Some lines were called "fixed" lines as they were a solid line and others were called "broken" lines as they were divided in half. It was this combination of broken and fixed lines that created sixty-four variations of the symbol known in the book as a hexagram.

One rainy night I threw my coins and did a reading. My luck fell onto the twenty-seventh hexagram—the symbol of nourishment. It was a reading that spoke to me as though it were written for me as my personal creed. I grabbed my jacket to wear over my pink sweatshirt of "The Powerpuff Girls," which I bought at a children's store, that was fit for a six-year-old. In those early days of recovery I wore a lot of children's shirts and sweatshirts with empowering girl cartoon images. I think they somehow comforted me and gave me a sense of personal power and innocence at a time when I felt vulnerable in an adult world. I snatched up my umbrella and ran to a tattoo parlor I had seen near our apartment, splashing in rain puddles in my colorful, glossy galoshes like a giddy child. I drew the hexagram that I wanted on a sheet of paper for the tattoo artist, lay down, and had it etched into the underside of my arm. *This is a commitment to myself*, I thought, *from this day forth, to do my best to make choices that will inspire my wellbeing.* I felt that I was on my way to a place called Nourishment.

Despite the spiritual nurturance that began to evolve in my life and the sustenance I had gained from following my meal plan, anorexia still gripped me. Because I hadn't yet started the real work in therapy, I hadn't really let go of anorexia. And as a result, I encountered one thing after another that brought me to my knees. My honeymoon was over. Anorexia had gate-crashed. A couple of months prior to landing in the United States, I had stopped drinking. Then, on my first night in our New York apartment, our flatmate had offered my sister and me a couple of beers to celebrate our arrival. I drank a quarter of the bottle. I was in control. A week later, I drank half a bottle, and soon I drank a whole bottle. Then it became two bottles of beer and a bottle of wine in one night. Soon enough I was drinking beer, wine, and shot after shot of tequila in succession. For a few nights a week I drank in moderation, thinking, *I can do this, I'm in control*, but every so often I would let it rip. I booze binged. It was because the food was going well that I drank—I was still addicted to being addicted. It was because my emotions were still festering beneath the surface that I drank—I was still full of the pain.

One night after work I went to a club with another waiter. I had already consumed three glasses of red wine before leaving the restaurant. We waited in line. The bouncer ushered us past the red rope. We pushed through the crowd to the bar.

"A shot of tequila?" my coworker said. "This one is on me." The bartender poured a double shot of gold tequila that flowed into a tumbler like syrup. Up until that night, I'd only been drinking beer and wine, and I had forgotten the reek of hard liquor, the temptation of liquid gold.

"Jesus!" I shouted.

"You can handle it," he said, and he slapped me on the back. Half an hour later, I was back at the bar. This time I reached into my own pocket to pay for another double. Then I headed back onto the dance floor. Then back to the bar. Then back to dance. The next thing I knew, I was in my own bed, naked except for my underwear. It was two in the afternoon. I did not know how I got there. I did not know what day it was. I jumped out of bed. The room swirled. I keeled over. My head pounded. I felt the puke rising in the back of my throat. I zigzagged around the room searching for my clothes, which were strewn all over the floor. I crawled around on my hands and knees and fumbled under tables and couches and rugs. My sister walked in through the front door carrying a bag of groceries. "What's going on?" she said, walking up to me.

"I can't find my glasses. I looked everywhere. I can't find my glasses."

"Jesus, you smell like a brewery!" She stepped back and waved her hand in front of her nose. "When did you get home? Where were you last night?"

"I don't know," I said, steadying my dizzy body against a wall. "I went to a club after work. I drank tequila. I don't know how I got home. I don't know what the hell happened. I could have been raped for all I know." I paced up and down and collapsed on the floor.

"Calm down," she said in a firm voice. "You would know if you were raped. You would feel it."

She lifted me off the floor and helped me to the bathroom. She filled up the bathtub and slid her hands under my armpits so I wouldn't slip while I lowered myself into the tub. "I don't know why you do this to yourself," she said, lifting my head up so it didn't sink underwater. Before passing out, I heard her add, "It just never ends with you."

She called the restaurant to tell them I had a virus and was too sick to come in. She hoisted me out the bath, dressed me in soft pajamas, and tucked me into bed. I slept until the following morning. As soon as I got up, I left the apartment and walked the city in search of my glasses. I retraced my steps, the forty or so blocks, from the club to our apartment just in case I had walked home and lost them along the way. I looked for memories of the night. Clues to my blackout. Along the way I came across a patch of dark green blades of grass with a low metal spike fence around it. I had a flashback of the same old-fashioned streetlamp that hovered above the grass. I remembered lying in the dark curled up on the grass patch and looking up at the dim streetlamp, waiting for the world to stop spinning. I stepped over the fence and kneeled down on the grass and swiped my hands across the ground. I did not find my glasses. But I touched the short metal spikes of the fence that surrounded the grass. Had my drunken skull landed on one of them, I would have lost a lot more than my glasses.

I knew that every time I took a sip of the first drink of the night, I made the choice to enter the realm of self-abandon, recklessness, and uninhibitedness—a space that was all too familiar. It was a place that for a decade I called home. Part of me was aware that getting drunk and blacking out meant that I was still using in order to block out my emotions. I had merely substituted grub for booze. Another part of me fought this thought. I read a book called *Addiction is a Choice* and told my sister I was cured. I would choose not to become intoxicated, I said. It was that simple. I had free will. I had a choice.

Soon after that incident, after living in New York for six months, we were asked to leave our SoHo loft apartment because our flatmate's lease had expired. My sister decided she wanted to leave New York and return to Cape Town. She wasn't happy at her job and wanted to pursue the relationship she had left behind at home. I decided to stay. I loved my job at the Italian restaurant, I was earning good money, and I still did not feel ready to return home to therapy. When my sister left, I moved into an apartment in Brooklyn with two flatmates.

A month later, I drank at the same club as before and blacked out again. But this time was different. Once I sobered up, I tried to piece together my recollection of the night. I had vague flashbacks and one vivid memory. I remembered that I sat at the bottom of some subway stairs and vomited at my feet. I held onto trashcans for balance. People crowded around me asking, "Is she okay? Is she okay?" I picked up the receiver of a pay phone to call a friend, but the numbers morphed in my mind and I could not catch them. Then I was on a subway car. I heard Times Square being announced. Then there was another subway. More vomit. More announcements. Then the train came to the end of the line. I came to. The only other person on the train was a Mexican guy with a moustache who was asleep with his head on my shoulder, snoring. I pushed his head off, stood up, and hobbled outside.

I do not know where I am, I thought, *or how I got here. I have no idea what happened last night.* I sat on a bench and looked up at the piercing morning sun. Snow melted on the ground. I patted myself up and down to feel if I had been assaulted—or just to make sure all of me was there. My scarf was wrapped around my neck. My shoelaces were done. My zipper was zipped up. I was wearing my clothes the way I would have gotten dressed in them. I pulled my gloves off. My hands felt muggy and wet with sweat. I shivered from exhaustion and cold.

What the fuck am I doing to myself? A woman in a neat black coat, pointy shoes, white gloves, and combed hair stood erect waiting for the next train on the platform. I asked her where we were and what time it was. We were far outside Manhattan in a borough I was unfamiliar with. It was just after nine in the morning. I knew I had left work at midnight. I knew I went to the same club where I had blacked out before. I knew the club closed at two in the morning. I knew I went there with the same waiter I had gone with before, this time to celebrate our earnings. I knew I had earned three hundred dollars the night before. I counted my money. It was all there minus forty dollars I must have used to buy alcohol. I realized I had spent seven hours riding different subways in my pathetic attempt to get home and all I had needed to do was hail a cab. But I was too wasted to think of it.

That was the last I drank for years. I knew that one more sip could get me killed.

I stayed in New York for another few months and began to experience a deep loneliness. I sat in my tiny windowless room with the radiator on full blast, drawing pictures of the sun. I felt like my higher power and all the people of the world had abandoned me. I was hurt and angry that my intoxicated fling with my Italian manager ended in rejection almost as soon as it began. Yet I was unable to access my deep pain. I did not connect what I felt with anything that was happening in my life. I just let the sadness scrape past me and continued the daily grind until my visa expired. I had had enough of anonymity. I decided I would take the money I earned and use it to fly home but then buy an open ticket around the world. My idea was to keep moving, to avoid going home to confront the feelings I had run away from my whole life.

On my return to South Africa, after one year in New York, I bought a ticket to Europe to visit the prince, whom I had not forgotten, and who was by then living in his hometown of Amsterdam. I wanted to see if he was really my true love. I still hoped and believed he was. And from there I would travel on to my dream place: the Amazon rainforest. A huge part of my motivation for traveling was that my sister had found freedom for her spirit when she traveled and she wanted the same for me and so encouraged me to do it. I convinced myself that it was the right thing for me and that, just as it had done for her, it would free my spirit and get me in touch with my true self.

"I will be gone for three years," I told my mom. "Not a day less."

"But you need to be here, to be rooted, to resume therapy and spend time with your family, the people who love you," she said. "You need to stop running away."

Although I ignored her plea, she convinced me to go to an alternative therapist before I left, a woman she had heard of who was known around town as a healer with shamanic powers. Her name was Katja, and when I went to see her, she tried to do bodywork on me, but I resisted. She tried to reach me on an energetic level, but apparently I blocked her. After all the spiritual seeking I had done in the past year, I still lacked the courage to do the real work. This of course would have included returning to Gregory for one-on-one therapy, rejoining my support group and checking in with Tracey around my meal plan. Instead, I gave both Gregory and Tracey a call to let them know I was going backpacking in Europe. Again, Gregory expressed his concern for my well-being and again I ignored his warning.

A couple of weeks later, my mom found me sitting cross-legged on the floor in her apartment, stuffing my clothes into a backpack.

"I thought Katja told you that what you need most is to stay put and be grounded," my mom said, clasping her hands behind her back and looking down, forlorn. "But yet again you are escaping. When are you going to stop?" Her voice sounded hopeless.

"My eating is on track, Mom. I've stopped drinking. And I'm not running away. It's called traveling. I can even visit your sister in London. It's just a short flight from Amsterdam. She'd love that. I haven't seen her in ages, and I know she'd love to pamper me."

"But don't you think it's enough now?" she asked, hovering over me as I zipped up my backpack.

I looked up at her quizzically and answered, "No."

My first stop was Amsterdam. The prince was at the airport to greet me. He had swapped his black leather pants for stiff bright blue jeans, and a jade pendulum hung around his neck. We embraced awkwardly and checked in with each other: How was New York? How is Amsterdam? Friends? Lovers? Soul mates? Strangers? Foes? I told him that soon after he left Cape Town, I had joined a support group. I told him I was now an anorexic in recovery. I told him I missed him. He told me that soon after he left he had met a girl. He had fallen in love and then split up. Now he was fucking someone else he had just met. He said he missed me. I wondered why he hadn't told me all this on the phone. But maybe he had—I probably had not wanted to hear it.

Later that day at his parent's home where he was living, he sat me down and looked into my eyes. We were sitting cross-legged on the cold stone paving in his parents' kempt Dutch garden facing each other, surrounded by pretty flowers.

"I need to tell you something important," he said. "I have done a lot of soul-searching, and I have found new meaning in my life. I am a spiritual seeker and Reiki healer now. My mission is to learn about my higher self. I am studying with a famous guru here in Amsterdam. Before you got here, I meditated and prayed long and hard on this, and I have finally come to a realization from deep in my soul that I am not in love with you."

My heart stopped. The energy drained out of my body. I held my breath. He finished by telling me, "You are not the one." Every feeling of hurt and rejection I had ever felt in my life surfaced in that moment. My stomach contracted, and I buckled over. The pain hit me in the core of my being, my center, which felt so battered and unworthy. Then it started to rip me apart inside. I had not yet learned how to contain my feelings or to hold them separate from my sense of self. I had no idea how to verbalize that his rejection hurt me. I did not know that I could be assertive enough to stand up for myself, to tell him that if only he had come to this realization sooner I could have saved hundreds of dollars on a plane ticket. Instead, this feeling, this anger and hatred, flooded my whole being. The pain got so bad, so big and uncontrollable, that I ran straight upstairs to my luggage.

But instead of packing up to leave Amsterdam, I rummaged in my bags for the pocketknife my mom had bought me for the jungle as a going-away present. I was to use the blade to chop branches, open tin cans, and cut fruit. I ran to the bathroom, locked the door, and took the blade to my skin and slashed. I cut myself over and over and over on the soft skin on the inside of my forearm and felt no pain as the tears gushed. I felt pacified. Lulled. Vacant. But I felt nothing inside as the tears streamed down my face. That terrifying feeling stopped. Only then did I stop cutting. And then I had another pain to deal with—one that I could manage, one I could control. I let warm water wash over the bloody gashes and patted my arms dry with toilet paper. *I am taking care of myself*, I thought. But I was really just nursing a temporary wound instead of heeding to the terrified cry of my emotions telling me to get out of Amsterdam, to go home, to return to therapy, and to stop running away from my feelings.

Later that day I took a train on my own into the city. It was a half-hour ride from the prince's village. I smoked joints, that luckily gave me the munchies so I was compelled to keep eating, and stalked the streets stoned and enraged. I hung out in the red-light district and watched sex shows. I shared one small motel room with five twenty-something backpackers I met in the street, sleeping next to one of the guys in a double bed. I did anything to not feel alone. I did not want to admit to myself that I had traveled all the way to Holland for nothing. I was determined to know why my prince had rejected me. Why I was not good enough. Why the pain was so big.

Days later, when my money ran out, I returned to the prince's village with a raging bladder infection. The prince took me in like a dirty stray cat and suggested I eat only watermelon, and nothing else, for three days as a detoxifying remedy for my infection. It was a big mistake for a recovering anorexic like myself. I was oblivious to the fact that I had unashamedly strayed from my healthy eating plan and that my watermelon diet could very likely induce a relapse.

I made the choice to stay because I wanted answers. I wanted closure. And I did not want to leave until I got both. I spent the days earning my keep. I ironed his father's shirts, as a favor to his mother. I filed his mother's paperwork, as a favor to his father. And I repainted his parents' room, as a favor to both of them. I cooked dinner for the family. And when the work was done, I sat on the couch and watched the prince take his female client with the "hot body" upstairs so he could practice his Reiki healing on her.

"I'm not fucking her," he said with a grin before following her upstairs.

Looking back, it was a really good example of how undeserving I still felt of any kind of pleasure and how I felt I needed to suffer still in order to gain. I could not just be there as a guest and enjoy. I had to earn it. And I could not leave. I had to endure. It was the pattern of my life. A few weeks later, I piled into the family car with his parents, grandparents, and sibling to spend the summer on vacation with them at their stone cottage in the south of France.

I gained strength out in the country, where I basked in the sun wearing teenybopper panties with the words "I heart me" printed on the front and a tiny bikini top and sneakers, soaking up holistic information from self-help books I found lying around the house. However, instead of using it to guide me back home where I essentially needed to be, I decided next to traipse through Spain with the prince. *Never mind that I am emotionally depleted and physically drained*, I told myself. *No matter how exhausted I feel, I will not turn down the opportunity to accompany the prince to Barcelona. Maybe there I will get closure. Maybe there I will find my answers.*

W hen you are out of your mind and halfway around the world begging a Casanova for your sanity, it is only a matter of time before you crash.

I spent three days and three nights in Barcelona and contracted lice and scabies. The prince and I stayed at a backpacker hostel off the main promenade on the city square. The dormitory squeezed in fourteen bunk beds draped with dirty socks, underwear, and damp towels. Next door the bar stank of spilled beer and sweat. Downstairs flamenco dancers, clowns, and jugglers performed in the square. On the first night, the prince wanted to party. I wanted to sleep. He wanted to smoke with the prostitutes, flirt with the drug dealers, and dance with the jugglers. I wanted to be tucked in bed by ten in clean pajamas, cuddling a fluffy toy. Instead, I lay awake at midnight curled up under a stiff sheet wearing pants that I used as a towel to dry my body after my shower. I used my backpack as a pillow, for safekeeping. I realized then that I wasn't going to get any answers from the prince.

The next night, after gallivanting aimlessly, the prince was out partying, and I lugged my heavy body back to the hostel. A guy with dry lips, freckled skin, and orange dreadlocks down to his elbows followed me. He wore patched quilt-like pants and a hippie shirt torn around the neck. He spoke broken English and latched onto me like a wounded animal. He asked me to hang out with him, and I wanted company, so I said yes. We tramped through the back alleys all night, hand in hand like young lovers. He wanted me to stay with him in Spain, marry him, and make a living like the two masked clown acrobats we saw juggling balls. And for a very brief moment I entertained his fantasy in my own mind. *It would make a great story*, I thought.

On the morning of the third day, the prince left me alone in Barcelona and returned to Holland. That was the last time I ever saw him. My throat closed. My stomach shut down. My head spun. I struggled to breathe. A panic around food that had barely visited me for almost a year and a half now breathed down my neck. It was an all-too-familiar reaction to feeling abandoned, alone, and unsafe. That day, I passed the same bakery again and again and eyed a small croissant in the window. I put my nose up against the glass to look at it. I saw the soft pastry dough. I smelled the butter. I could all but taste the crisp edges and the soft, buttery underbelly.

The saleslady at the till glared at me, so I stormed up the street, pacing, wringing my hands, hyperventilating. I walked and walked and looked in all the windows along the way at all the different food. Everything I saw posed a sort of life-or-death decision. Whatever I chose would determine my fate forever after. If this, then that. If that, then this. If this, then what? I returned to the same bakery, peered through the window, and eyed the same croissant. I wanted it. But my hands were tied. My tongue was twisted. My voice was gone. I could not bring myself to walk into the store.

Again, I paced up and down the street and begged myself to

make this small yet massive decision while being consumed by an overwhelming urgency to satiate the hunger and an equally powerful compulsion to quell it through resistance. For most "normal" people, something as mundane as buying a snack for breakfast would be a miniscule, transient, and irrelevant detail in the scope of a day. But to me, in those moments of panic and anxiety, the magnitude of such an overwhelming decision was everything and more. It was impossible. So I did not eat anything the whole day or night. My mind had snapped. The one thing I did buy was a children's T-shirt with a cartoon image of a little girl, which, just like the Powerpuff Girls sweatshirt that I wore daily in New York, felt strangely comforting and snug, especially at such a vulnerable time when I needed something to make me feel safe and held.

I am lost and scared, and I do not know how to make it better. Everything is too much. It's all too much. What is happening to me? Where is my mind? Where is my mommy? I'm fucked. I am going to die. I can't breathe. I can't swallow. My head is spinning. Where am I? How am I going to get out of here? Stop! Stop this! I need help. Help me. Help me. I am going down. I can't get out. My head is spinning. I'm going down. I'm falling. Save me. Please save me. Get me out. Get me the fuck out. I am going to die. I am going to die. I am losing my mind.

The child in me was terrified, and the adult in me had no idea how to make it better. I had not yet learned how to take care of myself in what to me was such a terrifying situation. I had no idea how to cope during a downpour of feelings of rejection, abandonment, aloneness, and loneliness. Even though I had only subjected myself to that "unsafe environment" for a total of three days, I was drowning in fear. I knew I was vulnerable, a child, incapable, irresponsible. I knew that I needed help. I pushed through the crowds and wandered around in a daze, apologizing in my broken Spanish for bumping into people. Hours later I passed an Internet café painted in bright orange. I went inside, got online, and emailed Gregory back in South Africa.

I can't eat, I wrote. *I think I may have relapsed. Please please please write back ASAP and tell me what I must do.*

That night I crawled into the hostel bunk bed and prayed that he would reply fast.

In the morning I leapt out of bed wearing the same clothes as the day before, and I ran to the Internet café to check my email. I took a deep breath and closed my eyes. When I opened them again, I saw that he had written back.

If you relapse, the most important thing is that you go immediately to somewhere where you feel safe and you get back on track as soon as possible.

I sighed with relief and bowed my head and thanked my higher power for answering my prayers. I logged off and ran to the restroom to think. The room had faux marble white-veined tiles on the walls and a huge square mirror with lipstick smudges and water stains. An ultraviolet light suspended from the ceiling made me look like the skeleton of a ghost in an iridescent white shirt. The UV lights were there to stop heroin addicts from shooting up because it made it harder for them to find their veins. I stared into the mirror at my fluorescent skin, my petrified face, and my T-shirt that shone like a full moon in the black of night.

It is only in times of weakness that I can hear my heart crying for me to listen. I have to go home. I have to deal with this pain that I have ignored for so many years. I know it is time. I need to admit this and to accept it and work toward it. I need to listen to my heart. It wants to leave Barcelona. It wants to talk this shit out. It wants to be free to move forward.

I knew in that moment, when my heart beat like footsteps

on a tin roof, that I had run so far and so fast that I had run out of choices. There was nothing left. I turned away from that mirror with a small sense of purpose and was thrust into a trance. My body led, and I followed. It was as though a huge force swept me up, like a second wind, and deposited me, backpack and all, at the Barcelona airport. I booked the last seat on the last plane of the day to London to stay with my aunt, my mother's younger sister, in what I knew would be a place of safety. With the last of my money I bought a sandwich, the first "meal" I had eaten in days. I sat on a bench for eight hours to wait for my flight, put my feet up, put my earphones in, and took a bite of my sandwich. I watched the world go by, closed my eyes, and made a wish.

I wish I had the courage to believe I was strong enough to travel further, brave enough to face the world, and responsible enough to handle whatever comes my way.

I landed in London in the early hours of the morning. Along with the other passengers on my midnight flight, I disembarked and checked through customs. My aunt was there to greet me in a coat, her white hands peeking out from under her sleeves and her flushed face pale. She and her husband stood still and waited patiently side by side, shoulder to shoulder, both of them with earnest expressions and pink cheeks. When they saw me pushing a trolley with my backpack thrown on top, they smiled and stepped toward me to hug me. Although she and my mom look similar, my aunt is the antithesis of my mom. She is organized, punctual, and straight—nine-to-five, breakfast at eight, dinner at eight, and normality in between. She was exactly what I needed to feel safe.

"Sorry I only called yesterday," I said. "Thanks so much for coming out this early to get me."

"It's just like you to arrive at two o'clock in the morning," she said.

"We wouldn't have expected anything different," my uncle concurred.

I hung my head low and followed them out of the airport into the gray cold. My aunt looped her arm in mine and led me to their car. An hour later, my uncle went to bed, and my aunt and I sat together at her neat kitchen table in her orderly kitchen. Napkins were packed in a napkin holder. Coffee mugs were lined up on the shelves next to teacups. Checked kitchen towels were folded next to the shining metal sink. Oven mitts hung over the stove bar. She poured boiling water in my mug for tea and laid a porcelain jug of milk beside it. I relaxed my shoulders, cradled the warm mug, and sighed with relief.

"You'll be sleeping in our room," she said. "We made the futon in the study into a bed for us. That way you can sleep all morning if you like and you won't disturb us when one of us needs to use the computer in the study. There is a sleep machine next to the bed so you can choose from six different calming sounds of nature, and if you need anything at all, help yourself. I'll show you where everything is."

I climbed into their double bed with two pillows on each side and an under-sheet folded over the duvet cover and tucked between the mattress and base like a hotel bed. I pulled the crocheted blanket up to my chin and fell asleep listening to the exotic sounds of tree frogs and crickets on a summer night in the tropical jungle that I never got to see.

I woke up later that afternoon. I opened my eyes and cried. The sleep machine played sounds of ocean waves whooshing onto the shore and back again, and I wanted to throw up. My aunt knocked on the door to see if I was awake and said that breakfast was on the kitchen table: freshly squeezed orange juice in a tall glass, lightly buttered seven-grain toast, a bowl of muesli, and a tub of organic strawberry yogurt.

"Coffee?" she asked as I sat down, the percolated roast filling the room. I nodded yes. The open door that led out to a small wooden patio let through a crisp wisp of air, and a soft ray of sun warmed my back. I slumped into the chair, and my stomach relaxed.

No more chasing, hassling, deciding, pondering, craving, searching, yearning, hunting. It is all here. Predictable. Safe. Orderly. This is the rehab I have longed for. This is it. This is the nurturing that I have needed all along.

My aunt, without even knowing it, had saved me from what could have been a heavy relapse back into the darkness. For the two weeks that I stayed at her "rehab," the same breakfast of muesli, yogurt, toast, and juice was laid out for me every day. I realized then that breakfast was the most important meal of the day to keep me in check emotionally. I called my bowl of muesli my "Medicine Bowl" after an American Indian tarot card I once read. *Some people have to take their morning pills*, I thought. *I have to eat my Medicine Bowl. Every single morning.*

On my second day in London I found a book on anorexia on my aunt's bookshelf. It was a simply written clinical self-help book with basic explanations and practical exercises. Even though Rob had given me his book, *The Unknown World Behind Eating Disorders*, I hadn't read it. So this was the first book I had ever read on anorexia. I went through it page by page and came across an exercise advising the reader to write her life story. So after breakfast every day, I sat in the gentle noon sun on the kitchen patio and wrote pages and pages of my life story on a lined yellow notepad. It was the first time I had ever written out every little thing chronologically and in detail. I wore hippie clothes from the sixties that my aunt was throwing out because the cloth felt soft on my skin. I felt like a modest pilgrim on her way to finding inner peace.

Every afternoon I wore a duffle coat to walk outside alone in the park near the house listening to Tibetan mantras on my Walkman. It was a soundtrack to a film about a Nepalese tribe who carry salt across the Himalayas in the snow. An epic journey. *All I am trying to carry is myself*, I thought, *and even that is too hard.* I hummed the chants on my walks, readying myself to return home and face the feelings I had been running from for what now seemed like forever. To face myself truly.

On my last day in London, I caught the tube to the city center and found myself in an artsy bookstore on a street corner. A box in the back of the store overflowed with second-hand paperbacks. I reached in and found a tiny book the size of my hand called *The Little Book of Happiness*. The book instructed its reader to close her eyes, put out her intention, and open the book to a random page, where her message would await her. I closed my eyes and opened the book onto a page that read: *Go home. Find freedom. Give it all your energy.*

"Therapy." That was my answer whenever anybody asked what I was going to do now that I was back in South Africa after my global sojourn.

"And?" they asked next.

"Therapy."

I returned to Gregory, whom I had abandoned just three months into our sessions. I didn't need to see Tracey because my food had been consistently on track, except for my relapse in Barcelona. In my first session back, I again sat opposite him in his yellow room. He wore the same bottle-green cardigan and lace-up brown shoes. His hair had grown longer on top, and his sideburns now had a gray tinge. I hadn't seen him in a year and a half, and I would have liked to consider myself a worldly explorer, a conqueror of nations from the Americas to Europe. Instead, I returned with a broken heart and a bumpy tale to tell. I grabbed a Kleenex from the plastic box and noticed next to it the only new addition to the room, a mini Zen sand garden with a tiny rake and three smooth pebbles—black, white, and gray.

I looked up at Gregory with my elbows slumped on my knees, the Kleenex dangling from my fingers. I knew he was aware of my journey and my failed plans. He was the one person I turned to not even a month before when I relapsed in Barcelona. I wanted him to tell me it was okay, that there was no reason to feel ashamed or like a failure. I wanted to hear that I was not bad and incompetent. I knew he could read the disappointment on my face, but still he waited for me to talk first.

"I know exactly what you are thinking," I said. "You are looking at me and thinking that I fucked up. I had planned, I had dreamed, I had wished to get to the jungle, but I didn't get there. I didn't make it."

"Is that how you feel?" he asked.

"There I was, thinking that I could do a jungle-survival course, but I could barely survive my day-to-day living!" I said, ignoring his question.

He dug his elbows into the armrests of his chair and leaned forward.

"Let me explain to you what happens when you begin your recovery. First, you regress to the age that you were when it all started—emotionally."

"So are you saying that I'm like a teenager, like I'm fourteen?"

"Well, what I am saying is that given the fact that you were unable to address your true feelings during the course of your disorder, that it is likely that your emotional growth has been stunted, which would result in an emotional immaturity. This would subsequently require that you be patient and kind to yourself while you take the time to allow yourself to do the growing up that you weren't able to do all those years so that you can work toward ultimately becoming an autonomous adult."

It was true that I was living at home again with my mom under her emotional and financial care like a twenty-five-year-old dependent teenager, but it was also true that I had saved enough money waiting tables at the Italian restaurant that I would soon put down a large deposit on an apartment in Cape Town that my family would help me to buy.

"Fine!" I said. "So what exactly am I supposed to do now?"

"You will need to do the work," he said, looking me straight in the eyes.

I decided I was finally ready to learn to become an autonomous adult.

The following week I was at another session with Gregory. He asked me how I was feeling and waited for me to answer. I told him that five years before, in the pit of my anorexia, shortly after my microdot acid trip, my uncle had loaned me the book *Siddhartha*, by Hermann Hesse. It is the story of a young man who dedicated his life to reaching enlightenment. It is the story of the Buddha. Yet his lifelong journey to reach that self-awareness began as what Hesse describes as "a temporary escape from the torment of Self." I had read it over and over from cover to cover. I had relished every word. I had copied excerpts from it into my journal and summarized every chapter again and again to make sure I had absorbed the lessons.

"Why do you think this book spoke to you?" Gregory asked.

"Because I identified with Siddhartha's journey," I said. "His path was one of torment and decadence and perseverance. He left home at a young age to live among the ascetics, and he learned to deny hunger, to fast, to endure pain, to hold his breath, and to renounce his body."

I felt a pain in my chest like a bruise and a lump in my throat.

"So," I continued, "what I've been thinking is that maybe my journey as an anorexic has been like Siddhartha's ascetic journey. Maybe it was all just a spiritual quest, to escape the torment of my Self."

"I don't think so," Gregory said. "One is an allegory, and the other is a disease."

"Maybe so, but both are about self-discipline and abstention, even though anorexia formed on an unconscious level."

"You cannot compare the two," he said, shaking his head from side to side and shifting his position in his chair.

"Well, I still think that on some level, my anorexia was a kind of ascetic quest."

In the following session I begged Gregory to let me go into the rehabilitation clinic even if just for a few sessions a week as an outpatient. I told him that I did not want to do it alone again and that it would not be fair of him to leave me alone out in the cold. He agreed to let me attend two mornings a week of life-skills sessions and art therapy.

The first day my mom dropped me at the clinic, I felt like a toddler attending day care. I walked into the room and sat in the circle on the floor. The girls ranged in ages from early teens to late twenties. I was twenty-five years old. The girl opposite me sat twirling her hair around one finger, the girl next to me picked at her foot, and a lot of them stared into space. The occupational therapist did roll call.

"Today we are going to talk about naming feelings," she said, looking around the circle of slouching, yawning, leaning girls.

"Just because a feeling doesn't have a name, it doesn't mean it isn't a feeling, right? In time we'll all learn to identify our feelings and to better express them. Okay?"

She stepped outside the circle to open a window.

"Now, I want each one of you to close your eyes and visualize how you feel in this moment, which means thinking of an image to describe your feeling, such as, 'I feel like I'm drowning,' or, 'I feel like I'm sinking.' Once you see it, open your eyes."

She wrote our responses on the whiteboard. One girl said she was stuck on a high wall, and another said she was falling into sinking sand, and I said I was floating on a small raft in a storm.

After we'd all shared what we were feeling, the therapist said, "Now imagine what each one of you would do in these situations. For instance, you might call for help or try to surrender or cry or scream. This is a really good technique that you can use to communicate if you feel too overwhelmed to think. Okay?"

By that stage, I had been in recovery longer than most of the girls, many of whom had relapsed. Some were severely underweight, and some were paralyzed by fear. I found out that one tall emaciated girl had recently been discharged from the hospital after she was confined to bed rest and fed intravenously. The doctors had given her two weeks to live unless she agreed to the refeeding and thereafter to be an inpatient in the rehab clinic. Another girl had been admitted to the clinic three times before and would be discharged in a few days' time because her insurance would not pay anymore. There was one girl who was leaving the following day because she had successfully completed the program and was set free to enter the real world. She clung to her friend and cried.

———

In between my sessions at the clinic I sat in my mom's apartment and behind closed doors did my homework for the week. I sat cross-legged on the rug with rainbow-colored crayons splayed out in front of me as I drew drawing after drawing, using my non-dominant left hand to bring out my inner child, of princesses with pink fairy wings and hearts and yellow daisies and bunny rabbits and fluffy clouds with funny faces and rainbows with no end.

One day, my father called.

"Where are you? What are you doing?" he asked.

"Drawing," I said.

"For what?"

"I'm doing exercises to help me get in touch with my inner child."

"Your what? Why are you wasting time with all this shit? There is no inner child! Don't you understand? In life, you grow up—"

"But—"

"No, no, listen to me. We are born, then we become babies, then children, then teenagers, then adults, and that is where you leave the child behind! In the past. The child is gone when you become an adult. I have been telling you for years that you have to grow up!"

I held the receiver away from me and clenched the speaker side in my hand and screamed into the phone, "That is what I am trying to do!" I slammed the phone down and burst out crying.

A few weeks later, my father agreed to go with me to therapy. Although we had had our brief bonding vacation together in New York, I still felt that our relationship was somewhat forced and corrupted. But I wanted it to change. I wanted so badly to have a good relationship with my father by the time I turned thirty. It was my dream.

The day we went to see Gregory together, we sat next to each other on the sofa, and Gregory asked his usual questions even though he knew very well why we were there and what I hoped to achieve. Then I heard my father talk, for the first time, about what actually happened to him in Israel and about why he had left the country so suddenly. He spoke softly, and I saw humility in his eyes that I had not seen before.

"I was in a very bad depression," he told Gregory. "My business was liquidated, and I lost everything. It was one of the worst times of my life. It was so bad that I could not even take care of myself, let alone my own daughter." He bowed his head to his chest as if he felt ashamed.

I understood, in that moment, that his rage had had less to do with me being unworthy and unlovable, and everything to do with his own inability to care for himself on every level. I realized he had had a breakdown and that I had just, unfortunately, been in his way. In that moment, I turned to face him and said, "I forgive you." I knew that our relationship would only get better. And it did.

Around that same time, during my life-skills sessions at the clinic, I learned a skill that would have been useful to me during my stay in Israel with my dad. It might even have prevented our fights and certainly would have softened the blows. We did role-playing skits where we acted out incidents that left us feeling violated in some way. One girl acted as the perpetrator and the other the victim.

"Every one of you has the right to say NO," said the therapist before we began the skits. She slammed her hand against the whiteboard. "You will slowly transform from a wounded child to a responsible adult by creating boundaries for yourself, and you will become assertive rather than passive or aggressive or passive-aggressive. The goal is for us to become assertive, which ultimately means verbally expressing what we want to say in a calm and sensible tone."

We stared blankly.

"All of you are so used to expressing your emotions through your bodies rather than expressing them through your words. But saying no to food, no to pleasure, no to life by starving your bodies does not serve you in any way."

During the role-play, some girls giggled, some refused to participate, and others acted as though it were real. We said the word *no* so many times that by the end of the session it was coming out of our ears.

"In time you will learn that you create your own boundaries, your own space around you, and that you don't need your anorexic body to do that for you. You will learn to ask for what you do and don't want. You will learn to stand your ground because you believe you are worth it, not because you are trying to defend yourselves."

In every session, we sat in a circle, and the therapist facilitated our processes. One day, we lay down flat on huge sheets of paper and traced outlines around one another's bodies, which we either attacked with pens and scissors or adorned with material and crayons. Each collage was meant to relate to our body image, our emotional pain, and how our self-perceptions had become so distorted through anorexia. Another day, we wrote letters asking our damaged bodies to forgive our cruel minds, which we stamped and mailed to our home addresses.

The exercises were simple, some even puerile. But they were designed to match what we could handle in our vulnerable states of mind. Most of us were raw and angry and volatile even in our apathy and silences. Although I had traveled and worked and tried to have meaningful relationships, a lot of the girls had been confined to the rehab clinic, their every move monitored, their rebelliousness punished with bed rest, their resistance met with no pity, their food calculated down to the last morsel. Many of their emotional states bordered on anarchistic. And the duration of one girl's illness matched the intensity of another's, and vice versa. I was one of the few who had been anorexic for ten years, whereas some girls had an acute onset with a rapid decline in a few months or a couple of years. Although our stories were different, our disorders were the same. We heard our own pain in one another's cries and saw our own fear in one another's bodies.

In addition to life-skills sessions and art therapy and private sessions with Gregory, I also attended the same support group as I had before—once a week, every week. It confirmed, once again, that I was not alone and that there were other girls in the room who saw the world just like I did. It gave me renewed hope that I would come to understand myself in light of my disorder with the help of professionals who could relate to the lunacy that is anorexia without judging me as insane.

One night, months down the line, I sat in the same circle of chairs with some of the same faces I had seen at my very first meeting two years before, when I had worn my little-girl outfit and had my wild orange hair and skinny body. By now my hair was back to its normal color and curl, my fleshed-out body was in fitted jeans, and I wore a long-sleeve top that covered my belly. I sat with my legs crossed and my hands on my lap, like an autonomous adult would sit. Gregory went around the room and asked each girl to share how she was doing. I heard a few of the regulars complain about the same things: "I feel fat." "I didn't follow my meal plan." "I'm using." When it was my turn I smiled and announced my two-year anniversary of recovery. I received congratulations and applause. Everyone said I looked so well.

"Anything you wish to share with us tonight?" Gregory asked, smiling.

"I would just like to say that it's amazing to get dressed in front of the mirror every morning without judging myself as fat or thin, or to have a bad day just because I am having a bad day and not to blame it on feeling fat."

For a long time, support group was the only safe space I could go to acknowledge the pain of my past while I presented myself to the rest of my new world as normal. And time after time I heard Gregory use the same words over and over again whenever he asked us to share how we were doing. Then one day I got it. I finally understood that my anorexia was my need to control my emotions. Despite its complexity and chaos and confusion, it was in essence nothing more. Only then did I really begin to wade through the layers and intricacy of the disorder and to learn to see it and understand it for what it is. I finally grasped what Gregory had said every single time he had asked us to share how we were feeling and our generic response had been, "I feel fat." "Fat is not a feeling," he had said, over and over and over again.

Fat is not a feeling.

Chapter Twenty

FORGIVENESS

There were only so many times that I could talk about feeling my feelings without actually feeling them, and there were only so many skills that the clinic could teach me; I'd have to figure out the rest in my own time.

I signed up for a six-month group-therapy workshop with Katja, the shamanic healer who my mom had taken me to see before I had left for Amsterdam. Katja lived an hour outside of Cape Town central, over hills and through valleys. Her home overlooked open fields and a hazy mountaintop. Her white house was a two-story clay abode, with a pebble path leading up to the door, high ceilings, and a fireplace. The living room doors opened out onto a garden with a sloping hill, a plastic wading pool, and thick lavender bushes planted in an all-purple flower garden. Purple is the color of enlightenment.

My mom and I vowed to take part in the workshop together, for one weekend a month, for a period of six months. We knew it would be our chance to reconnect and understand each other's pain of the past. We would share the space with four other women who we would come to know as clan sisters. One by one we would each succumb to a primal process and cry, weep, scream, dance, chant, beat pillows, and cradle each other like babies until we had nothing left inside. Katja would guide us through and protect us like a lioness would her pride. On our arrival, Katja was standing outside barefoot waiting to greet us, her arms adorned with wire and wood bracelets. A round stone pendant, her talisman, hung around her neck on a leather string, and her brilliant orange hair shimmered like koi fish scales. She stepped inside to welcome us into her home. She had moved all her furniture to one side of the room to make space for the group. All that remained in the living area was a bamboo rug, pillows, and the air of a sacred space full of secrets and promises.

Once everyone arrived, she asked us to find a comfortable seat on the pillows on the floor and to form a circle. Sun streamed in, and the wind blew gently, and I smelled the sweet scent of burnt kindling in the fireplace behind me.

"It is important for each one of you to heed to your own needs in this workshop," she said in a steady tone that sounded like a chant. "You will need to be aware of yourselves in every moment and respect one another's space and words. This workshop is a time for each one of you to get in touch with your deepest selves and to unblock the pain holding you back from fulfilling your divine potential in this lifetime."

She asked us all to hold hands and to honor our scared beings with a silent prayer. Then she spread out a deck of tarot cards facedown on the ground and asked us each to pick one that would guide us on our journey. I picked the card of integrity and held it against my chest. Katja went around the room and asked each of us to share with the group what our cards meant to us. When it was my turn, I said, "My card is about asking for guidance to learn to stand proud in who I am. More than anything in the world, I want to have self-worth."

Later that weekend, I told the group that the week before, I was in a session with my psychologist, and we were discussing sex. I told him that I could get any guy I wanted in to bed with me. Then I said to him, "I bet you that if I really wanted to get you in bed with me, I could." I didn't realize at the time that I was experiencing transference—a normal and healing aspect of therapy. I told the group that I only realized a few days later what my words really meant—that for so many years I had traded my self-worth for sex.

After I finished telling the group my whole history of boys and bruises, I broke down and cried. Katja told me to let it all out, to scream if I felt like it or beat pillows if I wanted to, to get it out of my body, to let it go. Katja sat still on her wooden stool. I screamed until I collapsed. I lay in a heap on the floor, my arms tense from pounding pillows, my throat hoarse from screaming, my body weak from exorcising. And I cried till I had no more tears. All the women in the room held the space still for me. They waited patiently for me to come back to the present.

"I feel violated," I said finally in a whisper. "I'm so angry with all these men. I don't know what to do with this feeling."

"If you want to move forward in your life, you will need to let go of all your resentments and take full responsibility for having allowed it," Katja said.

"But I didn't allow it," I retorted. I propped my body up on one arm and wiped my face with my sleeve. "All those times . . . I was not in my body. Some other girl possessed me—anorexia— and allowed me to feel raped. I had no control. I was not me."

I collapsed back onto the pillow and wept. *I was not me. I was not me. I was not me. I was not me.* The room buzzed, and I felt as though a torrent of water was poured over my head.

"You can say that over and over again, you can scream and shout and cry, but it won't change you deep inside," Katja said.

"If your intention is to be free of the shame and guilt and re-sentment holding you back in your life and causing you so much pain, then you are going to need to take responsibility for your actions regardless of which powers ruled you at the time. You will need to find forgiveness for yourself."

Katja sat back and folded her arms over her chest. Her bright orange hair sparkled in the sunlight. Her bangles sounded like wind chimes. My crying finally slowed and I said, "It's easy when you are drunk or high to blame your shame on the alcohol and the drugs. But it's hard to forgive yourself when the perpe-trator is you." I wanted her to wrap me up and cradle me in her earth-mother arms like a newborn baby. I wanted a man, any man, to sweep me up in his arms and embrace me. Instead, I crawled over to my mother, and for the first time in years, I al-lowed her to hold me. She wrapped me up and held me tight and rocked me back and forth as I sobbed into her heart. I cried over the guilt I felt for having abused myself, my body, with no remorse for so long. She stroked my hair and held me tight and whispered, "It's okay, it's okay, it's okay." I felt her body tremble and her hands shake, and she started to cry with me as we held each other.

Over the months that I participated in the workshop, I remained celibate and sober. I watched myself slowly transform into the young woman I wished to become, even if only superficially at first. I went from wearing sweatpants and sweatshirts to silky tops, flowing skirts, and earrings. I took up belly dancing and dedicated a new journal to discovering my sensuality, femininity, virginity, purity, fertility—in short, to my being a woman who knows her worth. I did an *I Ching* reading and received the hexagrams of returning (number twenty-four) and yin (number two). It symbolized that I was reclaiming my feminine side that was banished under anorexia's reign. And when acquaintances asked me what I was working on nowadays, I said, "Myself."

On the weekend of our penultimate workshop, we broke for a vegetarian luncheon feast and then stepped outside to Katja's garden to absorb some sun. I felt satisfied from my meal and tired from the day's emotions. I lay barefoot on the hot grass. The sun blared down, and I bent my knees to block it. I lay my hand on my soft skirt and felt the sweat from my forehead drip into my ears. Katja walked out from the kitchen wiping her olive-oil hands on her pants.

"This will be the last exercise of the day for all you beautiful women," she said.

Everyone moaned and said they were too tired and had no more energy. I sat up. Katja stood in front of us to demonstrate, blocking the sun with her broad body. Her shadow stretched far in front of her. A mountain view wrapped around her head like a turban. She widened her stance and stretched her arms out to the sides.

"I want all of you to find a spot on the grass—leave enough space so you don't bump each other—and stretch your legs and arms out wide to the sides like this, in Warrior Pose."

Slowly, everyone found their spots and copied her. I stood in the middle, surrounded by my female clan.

"Get comfortable in your pose. I want you to stand still and keep your arms outstretched. I don't want any of you to put them down until I tell you to."

Sweat itched my whole body, my skirt clung to my legs like seaweed, and my mouth was dry and thirsty. A couple of minutes later, I heard complaints from the other women: "This is too hard." "What's the point?" "I'm tired." "I'm thirsty." "I give up." One after another, the women fell to the ground like dying flies. I was the only one still standing tall with my fingers pointed outward like a bird's wings in flight.

You can do this. Keep going. You can do this. Don't give up. Push through. You can do this. You would do this if your life depended on it. Pretend that your life depends on it. Pretend. Pretend. Pretend.

My neck crawled, my feet ached, my jaw tensed up, and my stomach hardened to keep me standing. I shut my eyes to concentrate on the voice in my head, which was the only thing keeping me going. I made up my mind on that lawn like I made up my mind during my anorexia; nothing would make me give in. This simple exercise was symbolic of my life with anorexia. No matter how hard, how painful, how unbearable it was to be Ana, I endured it because in my mind, it was as though my life depended on it. It was that same willpower and desperation to survive that made me the last one standing on the grass that day.

Katja whispered in my ear, "You can put your arms down now. You can let go." I slowly walked my feet in until I stood upright like a tree. Stinging tears of gratitude streaked my cheeks as I lowered my arms to my sides.

I told myself, *I do not have to suffer anymore.*

Six months after our first workshop, our group congregated for our last weekend together.

Katja told us, "I want all of you to know that you have done a lot of the hard work, the painful regressive processes, the deep core stuff. I am so proud of you and honored to share this experience with you. Now go home tonight and acknowledge the arduous journeys you have undertaken and know that the hard work is done. It is now time to let go and celebrate. Celebrate the amazing, beautiful, strong women that you are. And tomorrow bring a gift to give to one another that we will all open together."

That night, I went home and looked up the word *celebrate* in the thesaurus. It gave these synonyms: *commemorate, observe, proclaim, broadcast, acclaim, praise, extol, venerate, honor, exalt, applaud, cheer, commend, revere, solemnize, hallow, consecrate, ritualize, bless, sanctify, glorify.* After reading the entry, I thought, *Not one of these words describes how I treated myself over the years.* Then I looked at the antonyms underneath all the synonyms: *ignore, disregard, overlook, condemn, despise, dishonor, profane, desecrate.* And I said to myself, *These words are all too familiar. I have had a deep, intense connection with each and every one of these words.*

That night I wrote in my journal:

No more. To the saboteur voice in me keeping me stuck in a degraded mindset. To anorexia, who said you do not deserve, you cannot have, you may not enjoy. To my father, who criticized me. To all the men out there who I allowed to trash my innocence. No more will I allow myself to be controlled by you! No more will I allow you to dominate my life! No more will I allow you to take what's important to me: my sanity, my happiness, my hopes, my innocence, my beauty, my confidence. These are mine! And I will own them!

The workshop the following day was dedicated to giving and receiving one another's gifts. When it came my turn to receive my mother's gift, she knelt before me and held out a bundle of bottle-green Indian cloth with tiny rose-colored ink stains and a folded letter. She had purposefully cut the cloth into strips of different lengths and widths and then retied the strips to create a bundled ball of cloth. She held it with her bottom hand face up and her top hand facedown. She passed it to me carefully and smiled expectantly.

"Each layer of material symbolizes the painful journey you have been through," she told me.

I looked at her face in pain, in love. She sat forward and leaned toward me on her haunches, both palms pressed onto her knees, waiting for me to discover my gift. I began to untie the knots and peel off the layers of strips and unfold the material. My shoulders tensed up, and my stomach contracted. I felt winded in my gut. The room was so quiet I wanted to scream. A pain that took over my entire being welled up inside me. The pain of unfolding the cloth was the pain of slowly letting love in and opening my heart again to my mother, to nurturance, to love. My mother's gift touched what I had worked so hard to protect. Her letter to me read: *Unravel. Inside you will find something precious.*

Inside, I found a small round mirror that fit in the palm of my hand. I held it up to my face and in seeing myself with new eyes, I caught a glimpse of something, someone, precious.

Chapter Twenty-One

LETTING GO

One month later, I had a dream. I was cradling an emaciated girl with bleached blonde hair and a body so weak it surrendered into my arms like a baby bird with broken wings. I held her tiny hands and gently felt her fragile fingers. I whispered to her that she was dying. There was no sadness, just a freedom of letting go, giving in, surrendering. I woke up from this dream, at three in the morning, with a strong sense that the dying girl was my anorexic self.

I woke up, and I began to write.

Epilogue

———

The other night I had a dream, the only dream I've had about anorexia in fifteen years since the dream that seeded this book. In this dream there was an art gallery with chapel high ceilings and white walls—a space so huge and so empty that it swallowed silence. Someone was crouched low, curled up in a fetal position, pressed up against a wall, scribbling on it with a ballpoint pen—scribbling hundreds and thousands of tiny words and sentences, all crammed together like an army of blue ants trying to take up as little space as possible in the enormous, empty white cube.

When I woke up, the symbolism of the dream was clear to me. During my anorexia, the writing in my journals looked just like that—tiny, crammed, jumbled, and barely legible. Just as in those days I made myself—my body, mind, and emotions—small, so too did I write small—all a sad, grave attempt to take up as little space in my life as possible, believing I wasn't worthy of taking up more. Author Marianne Williamson's beautiful words say it all: "Our deepest fear is not that we are inadequate. Our deepest fear is that we are powerful beyond measure. It is our light, not our darkness, that most frightens us. We ask ourselves, Who am I to be brilliant, gorgeous, talented, fabulous? Actually, who are you *not* to be?" It took me a decade and a half of healing once I started recovery to get that—who am I not to be? Now my body, mind, and emotions take up so much space that they fill my life, and my writing in one copy of this book alone uses eighty-five thousand words and takes up nearly three hundred pages of space.

I now look back and see my anorexic life as a faded photograph; the memories are there, but the feelings, the visceral experiences of that reality, have vanished. And in their place is my life as it is now, big, and in full color. Today I can say with all my heart that I am a woman in love with her life, in love with her body, in love with herself. Today I am a mother and a writer. I have a career, a dedicated yoga practice, and outlets for my creativity. I have healthy relationships with family and friends and I live each day at ease in my body and in my heart.

But it wasn't always like this. Don't think for a second that life has been easy since I started recovery. It took many long, hard years to learn to love myself. When I began my healing journey at age twenty-four, I committed myself fully to my recovery and forged ahead, suddenly carrying the full weight of my emotions. I began writing for publications as a self-taught freelance journalist in Cape Town although I struggled to earn a living and support myself as an autonomous adult. I had back-to-back relationships with men—some kind, some weak, some cruel—none of whom mirrored the worthy self I was fighting for.

At the time, aside from having begun to write this book and wanting to publish it, I yearned, more than anything, to birth a baby, to become a mother, yet I was still, on an emotional level, a child myself. I was still cutting to quell my pain, and, like my mother, I was diagnosed bipolar, due to mood swings and depressions, even though this later turned out to be a misdiagnosis. For many years I endured dark depressions. Gregory, my psychologist, said that only once I dealt with all the other emotions that arise when you let go of anorexia like anger, guilt, and shame, would I reach the emptiness inside. One particularly dark depression landed me in a psychiatric clinic for nine days on heavy doses of antidepressants and antipsychotic medication just a few months after I turned thirty.

Four months after I was released from the clinic, I reconnected with a long-lost childhood friend, who was living in America, and, after twenty-one years apart, I moved to America, got married, and started trying to conceive the child I so desperately wanted while I poured blood, sweat, and tears into finally birthing this book. What followed was the agony of immigration, of losing my previous life and family in South Africa, which hit me like a death; the struggle of a new marriage founded by two wounded friends; the darkest night of my soul experienced as a psychotic break while on a cocktail of misprescribed medication; the rehashing of shame and trauma in the rewriting of this book; and two years of infertility, during which I felt life was not worth living without being able to conceive my own biological child—which I finally did, naturally and without intervention. This was followed, a couple of years later, by a life-threatening ectopic pregnancy, which resulted in the loss of a much-wanted second baby; the subsequent fall of a marriage that had triggered every single raw wound of my past until I accepted the truth that we are better off as friends and coparents and we got a divorce; and, most recently, the news that my father was diagnosed with terminal lung cancer and given one year to live.

But despite all this, I have never relapsed, and I consider myself fully recovered from anorexia—her spirit has left me.

I write all this not as a victim or a survivor but to show that life goes on after anorexia. My mother was right when she quoted M. Scott Peck's first line of his book *The Road Less Traveled* —"Life is difficult." But it is also so much more than that. Now, at forty, I love my life. I love being a mother to my five-year-old son, the love of my life, and raising him in the Bay Area of California with communities of like-minded, conscious souls. I value and respect his father as a co-parent and lifelong friend who helped me release my wounded self. I enjoy my day job as a copywriter and blogger. I relish food, cooking, and eating, and it's so not an issue that I almost forgot to mention it. I cherish my yoga practice, which continually brings me back to my highest self. And I adore being in my body, feeling sexual, sensual, and free of shame, all of which created fertile ground for me to finally attract a beautiful man who mirrors the self-esteem I worked so hard to earn.

Recovery really is all about fattening up your self-esteem, empowering your sense of self, and learning to love yourself. When I first woke up to the idea of self-esteem as a force that propels you toward self-love, it was too abstract to comprehend. Now, I see self-esteem as a powerful energy that, as Caroline Myss, author of *Anatomy of the Spirit*, says, resides in your third chakra and becomes "the dominant vibration in our development during puberty." Myss writes: "The third chakra, often called the solar plexus, is our personal power center, the magnetic core of the personality and ego. The illnesses that originate here are activated by issues related to self-responsibility, self-esteem, fear of rejection, and an oversensitivity to criticism." All of these are classic anorexic struggles. Myss writes: "The third chakra embodies the sacred truth *Honor Oneself* . . ." and this is exactly what life after anorexia is all about—learning to honor yourself.

I am deeply grateful to be alive today and to have reached this stage of my life when I can finally say I am an autonomous adult. I am a woman who knows her worth. I stand proud in who I am.

Thank you for sharing my journey.

ACKNOWLEDGMENTS

For many years, the process of writing this book was, like ano-rexia, mine alone. However, it's impossible to go through recovery alone. I am so excited that after more than a decade of working on various drafts of this book, the time has finally come to thank all the people without whom I would probably not be alive today, let alone happy and healthy.

First, I want to thank Graham Alexander for holding my hand, gently and reassuringly, as I took my first steps on the journey of recovery. Thank you for all the incredible work you have done for anorexics over the years. I was so lucky to find such a gentleman. The support group you offered was my saving grace, the cornerstone of my recovery. Thanks to all the girls and women who shared their stories in group and listened while I shared mine. Special thanks to the anonymous woman, whose name I don't recall, who asked me how I healed. You could not have known that you planted the seed for this book.

Big thanks to Tanya Burger for your warm, personable ap-proach. You made it possible for me to trust you from the start. Recovery would not have happened without you or my meal plan. I am very grateful to Ron Heyman for first breaking my denial and then ever so diplomatically handing me the piece of paper that changed my life and led me on the path of recovery. Thank you for giving me hours of your time and for truly caring.

To Dr Ruth Bloch, thank you for your wise simple question and holistic thoughts on anorexia. Your invaluable insight opened the way to the self-forgiveness that was the beginning of my true healing. And thank you Kate Martiny for holding me with your ever-nurturing earth-mother energy and helping me to learn the greatest lesson of all: to stand proud in who I am.

You are a powerful, passionate healer. You changed my life. Thanks to Janet Earl for sharing your deep knowledge of anorexia and for encouraging me to think of recovery as empowering my sense of self. To David Jacobs, thank you for ten years of teaching me yoga and in so doing offering me a solid foundation for my lifelong practice. Two decades later, yoga continues to be my savior.

I am forever thankful to Franny Rabkin. You were the best friend a girl could ever wish for. I thank you with all my heart for standing by me and loving me even while I was falling apart. Thanks to Zvia Brumer for welcoming me into your home like a daughter. Your generosity knows no bounds. You were my home away from home. Thanks to all my friends along the way who read early drafts of my manuscript and gave me feedback: Linzi, Carla, Sabrina, Pia, Nathalie, Helen, and Deborah. And thank you, Anna, for hiring me at Pepe, where I got to eat the best food in New York City, every day, and for unexpectedly becoming my lifelong friend. This book is also in memory of Kate.

Thanks to sweet Rossy and Jeff for lovingly creating the most comforting environment for me at a time when I desperately needed it. And thank you, Jeffrey, for your writerly advice. Thank you, Hally, for giving me *Siddhartha* to read, which was the first positive thing I connected with in six years. It allowed me to open my heart to myself and realize the spiritual side to my journey.

To my dearest Gaggi and Den, I am the luckiest granddaughter in the whole world to have had you both in my life, all my life. Thanks for your excellent editorial suggestions, your absolute belief in my writing, your continuous support of this project, and, mostly, for your unconditional ever-loving, ever-caring nature. I cherish you.

I am forever grateful to my sister, Tal, for always catching me when I fall. You are my guiding light, a dewdrop. Thank you for your eternal love and kindness. You have been my mother and my best friend, but most of all you are my soul sister. I love you. Thank you for believing in my writing and for always knowing I could do this. Thank you also for blessing me with Elah and Eva. I love you both with all my heart. And Shawn, patriarch and Papa Bear, thank you for teaching me to take responsibility for my own happiness.

To my mother, Arlene Amaler-Raviv: You have loved me and stood by me forever, no matter what. Thank you for empowering me with your artistic talent, for nurturing the writer in me, and for reading almost every draft of this book. You are the most amazing woman I know, the best artist in the world, and my very own mother and friend. I love you with all my heart and soul.

Daniel, you are and always will be my daddy. I love you deeply, more than you can know, and all is forgiven. Thank you for your unflinching support of my writing and for your constant push to see this book in print. You have been an amazing source of encouragement and are still my number one fan.

To Michael, thank you for being the father of my child and lifelong friend. Thank you for your enormous support of this project in its early days. Your comments were invaluable.

And to my son, Lev, just as your name means "heart" in Hebrew, you are leading the way. Thank you for coming into my life and choosing me as your mother. I am blessed. I would also like to thank Katherine Boyle for encouraging me, sincerely, to persevere with this project. Your generous feedback and kind words kick-started the rewrite of this book. Many thanks to Elizabeth Crane for your stellar editing and valuable comments of the first draft. And enormous gratitude to Linden Gross, an amazing writing coach, for helping me transform my raw manuscript into what it is today. Linden, you understood me and my project better than I could ever have hoped for. The six months we worked together was one of the hardest periods in my life, but without your unwavering acumen and your persistent guidance, I could not have done it.

Last, but not least, I wish to thank Brooke Warner, my publisher and founder of She Writes Press for this incredible opportunity to give my book a second wind with a reputable press dedicated to women writers. Thank you for seeing the merit in my work and for helping me breathe new life into my book. I am truly proud to put this version out into the world. Thanks also to my project manager Lauren Wise for guiding me along every step of the publishing process and Julie Metz for designing a cover that I love. And to my publicist, Eva Zimmerman, I could not be more grateful to have you representing this work. Thank you for 'getting' me, for believing in my book, for seeing it as a force, and for giving it wings.

ABOUT THE AUTHOR

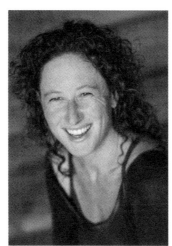

Shani Raviv is a published writer, writing coach, copywriter/content producer, and speaker who was born and raised in South Africa. She disputes the belief that an anorexic mindset is a life sentence and considers herself fully recovered. She lives in the Bay Area of California with her son.

SELECTED TITLES FROM SHE WRITES PRESS

She Writes Press is an independent publishing company founded to serve women writers everywhere. Visit us at www.shewritespress.com.

Learning to Eat Along the Way by Margaret Bendet. $16.95, 978-1-63152-997-9. After interviewing an Indian holy man, newspaper reporter Margaret Bendet follows him in pursuit of enlightenment and ends up facing demons that were inside her all along.

Not by Accident: Reconstructing a Careless Life by Samantha Dunn. $16.95, 978-1-63152-832-3. After suffering a nearly fatal riding accident, lifelong klutz Samantha Dunn felt compelled to examine just what it was inside herself—and other people—that invited carelessness and injury.

Insatiable: A Memoir of Love Addiction by Shary Hauer. $16.95, 978-1-63152-982-5. An intimate and illuminating account of corporate executive—and secret love addict—Shary Hauer's migration from destructive to healthy love

A Different Kind of Same: A Memoir by Kelley Clink. $16.95, 978-1-63152-999-3. Several years before Kelley Clink's brother hanged himself, she attempted suicide by overdose. In the aftermath of his death, she traces the evolution of both their illnesses, and wonders: If he couldn't make it, what hope is there for her?

Searching for Normal: The Story of a Girl Gone Too Soon by Karen Meadows. $16.95, 978-1-63152-137-9. Karen Meadows intertwines her own story with excerpts from her daughter Sadie's journals to describes their roller coaster ride through Sadie's depression and a maze of inadequate mental health treatment and services—one that ended with Sadie's suicide at age eighteen.

Raising the Bottom: Making Mindful Choices in a Drinking Culture. $16.95, 978-1-63152-214-7. Women share their drinking stories of hitting rock bottom—so you don't ever have to.